J

The Pregnancy Experience

THE PSYCHOLOGY OF EXPECTANT PARENTHOOD

The Pregnancy Experience

THE PSYCHOLOGY OF
EXPECTANT PARENTHOOD

Dr. Elizabeth M. Whelan

HARVARD SCHOOL OF PUBLIC HEALTH

W·W·NORTON & COMPANY

New York   London

Library of Congress Cataloging in Publication Data

Whelan, Elizabeth M
  The pregnancy experience.

  Bibliography: p.
  Includes index.
  1. Pregnancy—Psychological aspects.
2. Childbirth—Psychological aspects. I. Title.
RG560.W48   1978   618.2'001   78–15397
ISBN 0–393–01179–8

1 2 3 4 5 6 7 8 9 0

For Steve,
For Christine

Contents

Contents

Acknowledgments

The conception, gestation, and delivery of this book involved a large number of individuals whose professional interests, descriptions of their personal life situations, and attitudes toward childbearing proved invaluable in my research into the psychological aspects of pregnancy.

I gratefully acknowledge the help of Judith Nolte, editor of *American Baby;* Elisabeth Bing, author and childbirth educator; Dr. Amy Miller-Cohen, cofounder of Pondering Parenthood, a preparenthood counseling service; Molly McGrath of *Baby Talk;* Barbara Brennan, Chief Nurse-Midwife at Roosevelt Hospital in New York City; Rhoda Weyr, my agent, with William Morris Agency; and the more than two hundred and fifty men and women who offered their experiences and commentaries on the joys and sorrows of expectant parenthood.

Three people merit very special thanks: June Miller, my friend and assistant, who devoted many hours to each of the stages of this work—setting up interviews with parents and prospective parents, helping me locate research material, offering her own perspectives as a mother, critically reviewing—and then typing—all drafts. Steve, my husband, whose contributions of insight, patience, understanding, and encouragement spurred me on. And our daughter, Christine Barrett Whelan, who played a leading role in our personal pregnancy experience, and made us forever grateful that our answer to the question "A Baby? . . . Maybe" was "A Baby? . . . YES!"

INTRODUCTION

Why a Baby, Why a Book

My husband and I dealt with the question of parenthood much the way most intelligent, educated, career oriented couples do today. We ignored it.

Oh, the topic came up occasionally in the first years of our marriage (when we were in our mid- and late twenties). For example, when we would head to the shore for vacation, we'd look at the jam-packed back seat of our car, shake our heads and say, "Guess there's no room for a baby!" And as my thirtieth birthday approached, I would sternly announce to my husband, "We really must talk about the baby issue sometime soon—like this weekend." He would agree. But then the weekend came and went without a word said on the subject.

The whole question of having a baby was for me—and, as I subsequently learned, for millions of other women—a very emotionally unsettling one. Books like *The Baby Trap* (Ellen Peck), *Mother's Day is Over* (Shirley Radl), *The Case Against Having Children* (Anna and Arnold Silverman), countless magazine articles which revolved around the theme "none is fun," and literature from the National Organization for Non-Parents (NON) had informed us that parenthood was a drag, a sure way to terminate career plans, a possible threat to our marriage, an expensive, thankless job which would aggravate the Inevitable Population Explosion.

"Why invite disaster?" one part of me asked. But another part nagged, "You're not getting any younger. Motherhood couldn't be all that bad; maybe you'll regret it if you don't have at least one child . . ."

I am a rational, organized, plan-ahead type person. And I certainly didn't want to be accused of having a baby for any of those dumb reasons that Planned Parenthood and other such groups featured on bus and subway posters. I most definitely didn't want to bring a new life into the world until I was absolutely sure I wanted to be a mother, and thoroughly convinced that my husband was wildly enthusiastic about becoming a father. As my thirtieth birthday arrived and I felt as nervous as a turkey in November, I sought resolution of my quandary, approaching the question in the only way I knew how—scientifically.

I turned to hundreds of medical journals and psychological texts to find out why people have children, and to see how these reasons squared with my own current feelings. I intensively interviewed hundreds of couples to find out why they had children, seeing if I could sift the "right" from the "wrong" reasons. I talked with dozens of psychiatrists and psychologists to get their thoughts about why some people were so undecided about becoming parents, why others were sure of their feelings. And I turned my research into a book (*A Baby? . . . Maybe*), providing some guidance for what I called "the most fateful decision of your life."

Then one day it finally occurred to me that while the research I had done was invaluable, had allowed me better to understand the nature of the question I was dealing with, and had given me an opportunity to work through my dilemma, reading a dozen more articles or doing fifty more chi-square tests was not going to help. I had all the facts I could get. So I put away my calculator, slide rule, and balance sheet. And I turned to the question again, this time not as a scientist, but as a woman. And I found my answer. I simply wanted to have a baby.

What exactly did the word "want" mean for me? If I went into too many details here, I'd be anticipating the discussion I have in Chapter 1 on the "whys" of parenthood. But, in brief, my decision to have a child was based on a desire to experience what for so many couples is a major life event—to create a family unit and perhaps, in the process, to grow myself, embrace joys and face challenges I otherwise would never know.

Once The Decision was made, I thought the psychological turmoil would cease. But instead it intensified.

The first jolt I had after making up my mind was that I wasn't absolutely sure the decision was either firm or "right" for me. I continued to have second thoughts, a condition which violated my earlier set of rules for judging parenthood potential. I simply drifted one day from being 51 percent against having a child to being only 49 percent against it. Even without my calculator, I could tell the balance was a precarious one. Was I going to be able to keep my career intact and be a good mother too? Was this really the best time to have a baby?—so much seemed to be happening in our lives. Would we have to move to a new apartment? Or buy a house? How would we react to the responsibilities of a completely dependent human being? Frequently, the questions and new feelings of doubt nearly overwhelmed me.

The second preconception, postdecision jolt I received was that it was *I*, not *we*, making the decision. Again, I had previously convinced myself that if we were to have a child, my husband should be as eager as I about this most shared of all undertakings. But in reality he was still very hesitant. He was not totally against the idea (if he had been, this would have been a very different situation) but as far as he was concerned, life could go on forever the way it was. (I am happy to report now that our daughter is the joy of both our lives.)

Hesitant, still ambivalent, and not yet in full agreement on the subject, we began our pregnancy experience. During those 240 days (counting from when we got the news of the positive test), we both experienced the full gamut of emotions. During those months there were some very low points. Many of our expectations about pregnancy and parenthood were shattered, many of those romantic notions about having a baby were badly tarnished.

But there were some unexpected high points too. Thrills, anticipations, excitement which we could never have predicted. We were overjoyed and depressed, sometimes within the same hour. We found that other people began to react differently toward us, that our relationship with each other began to change. We started to see ourselves as different people, with new priorities and new roles in life.

We were not prepared for this type of psychological upheaval and, in an attempt to deal with it, sought help in books. But the books disappointed us because they focused almost exclusively on the physical aspects of pregnancy. After going through five or ten of the basic volumes for expectant parents, we began to feel that we knew more about the Fallopian tubes, progesterone, and cervical dilation than we really cared to.

The Pregnancy Experience is an attempt to fill the gaps in understanding the psychological events of pregnancy and those occurring immediately before and after it, to give you a frame of reference for evaluating and coping with many of those "normal crazy" feelings you will be experiencing for the next few months. It is not meant to be an all-inclusive book on the subject of pregnancy. It does not go into great detail about the reproductive physiology involved in having a baby, nor does it enumerate all possible medical complications of these nine months (you can find that in dozens of other books). Its primary emphasis is on the psychological experience of the *first* pregnancy (thus, for example, it does not deal at length with the question of the psychological impact of later pregnancies on the first- and later-born children), although it is clear that much of the discussion here will be appropriate for any expectant parents, regardless of family size.

Each chapter is divided into "psychological" and "physical" sections, discussing in the latter category only those physical aspects of pregnancy which are closely related to the expectant parents' anxieties, doubts, and general concerns; for example, making love during pregnancy, preparation for childbirth, and the decision of whether or not to breast feed.

I've written the book from two vantage points—as a woman who has recently undergone a pregnancy experience, and as a public-health scientist who has reviewed the available medical, psychological, and sociological information on pregnancy. I drew my material both from scientific sources (I avoided some of the more bizarre psychoanalytic material on pregnancy—for example, those which claim the primary motivation of a woman for pregnancy is to incorporate and retain the penis, resolving the final phase of a woman's phallic stage of development), and, more important, from talking with more than 250 couples—those who were planning a pregnancy, who were currently expecting a child, or who were already parents. I found some of these couples in childbirth preparation classes, in group childcare centers, in parks, playgrounds, elevators, subways, and department stores, and had the opportunity to talk with others who sought preparenthood counseling through A BABY? . . . MAYBE SERVICES℠, a New York City–based organization I established to counsel couples who face dilemmas and questions about parenthood—for example, about whether or not to have children.

I do not claim to have found a representative sample of American parents and prospective parents. Rather, I have incorporated the experiences of these men and women into my discussion of the psy-

chology of pregnancy as a means of lending some down-to-earth examples—optimally, some with which you will closely identify. I
must add here that not everyone I asked to talk with me about his or
her pregnancy experience was eager to do so. "Ohmygawd—I don't
even want to *think* about that subject!" was the response I received
from a number of parents, their reaction indicating that perhaps it
was an uncomfortable topic, reviving unpleasant memories—or
perhaps they thought just talking about it would be enough to initiate the reproductive process again.

In preparing this work, I started with six premises. First, that you
are now either considering the possibility of becoming pregnant,
wanting to get an idea of "what it's like" before you conceive, or that
you are now pregnant and plan to proceed with your pregnancy.
You undoubtedly have some doubts, reservations, second thoughts;
you may be frightened about the prospect of becoming a parent in a
matter of months. But I am assuming that you are not considering
terminating it. This book is not meant to counsel on the question of
whether or not to have an abortion.

Second, that the mental scars resulting from an unpleasant pregnancy experience can persist long after the episiotomy has healed.
You *can* learn to enjoy your pregnancy—and that means both of
you—and you *can* avoid the type of low points, arguments, and self-
doubts that can remain in memory long after your baby is born.

Third, that the most powerful elements that interfere with a
happy, normal psychological adjustment to pregnancy are fear and
misunderstanding: for example, fear of loss of your individuality;
loss of your spouse's time, love, and affection; the possibility of a
deformed child; misunderstandings about the nature of evolving
new relationships with others, about the expected emotional ups
and downs, about pain and discomfort in labor and delivery, and
about your new image as a mother- or father-person.

Fourth, that while all pregnancies are different (your life circumstances, age, whether or not the baby was planned, the birth order,
and other factors distinguish them), each represents a type of life
crisis, a sharp deviation in the normal course of events in your life.
The late Dr. Grete L. Bibring, a Harvard psychoanalyst who intensively studied first-time pregnant women some years ago, concluded that pregnancy is a "normal developmental crisis in the life

cycle," a time when you are moving irrevocably into another phase of your life.

Pregnancy is not just a static nine-month period of waiting. Having a baby is far more than simply conceiving and giving birth. The forty-week pregnancy period has its own unique conflicts, needs for adjustment, general reorientation of your life activities and goals. Even if your pregnancy was both carefully timed and very much wanted, it's a time during which you may experience happiness, fear, joy, resentment, fulfillment, physical well-being, physical misery, any feeling you can imagine. While a baby is being created physically, a family is being formed psychologically. Pregnancy represents the type of life crisis which, if favorably resolved, can benefit both of you, leading to greater maturity and self-esteem, resulting not only in the birth of a new child, but also in the birth of a number of new, healthy relationships.

Fifth, that this crisis affects two people very intimately: both the expectant mother and the expectant father. Too often, the pregnancy experience leads the woman to become increasingly concerned about herself and her body, while the man stands by wondering and worrying about exactly where he fits into this picture. *Both* prospective parents undergo a pregnancy experience. And, although for ease in writing, this book is directed toward the expectant mother (it is logistically difficult to write about psychological-physical topics in a way which is appropriate for both sexes), the nature of the material is such that it should interest both of you.

Sixth, that the pregnancy experience of the late 1970s and early 1980s may well be more tumultuous, characterized by more anxiety and conflict, than the pregnancy experience of earlier years. Not only are fewer women having children, but your ambivalence about becoming pregnant may be increased in knowing that when pregnant you can feel very different, quite conspicuous, and by the fact that today parenthood is a choice, one which is vying with other attractive options. In comparing my discussions about pregnancy with couples who are now in their fifties with those who have been pregnant more recently, I got the distinct impression that the modern pregnancy experience is a more emotionally trying one.

I organized the material in this book in a type of chronological order which I hope will parallel your interests as your pregnancy advances. A number of books for prospective parents have early chapters dealing with subjects which are of absolutely no interest to a man or woman in that stage. During months one and two of pregnancy, you probably are not all that interested in postpartum depression, nor would you really be eager to learn in an early chapter (as one book I reviewed assumed you would) about how to give a baby an enema. *The Pregnancy Experience* proceeds stage by stage, raising topics at points when they are likely to be of interest to you (for example, I am assuming that your interest in planning the type of labor and delivery you want will be in mid-pregnancy, not during your ninth month).

My purpose in writing this book is to provide you with information, comfort, assurance, and perspective, so that you might avoid many of the unsettling effects of aloneness, despair, and conflict, and emerge from your own pregnancy experience with a sense of both reward and exhilaration.

Elizabeth M. Whelan
New York City

The Pregnancy Experience

THE PSYCHOLOGY OF EXPECTANT PARENTHOOD

CHAPTER 1

Before the Fact

THE PSYCHOLOGICAL

Why Do You Want to Have a Baby?

First comes love. Then comes marriage. Then comes a baby. Maybe.

You are perfectly happy, your life is in equilibrium, your marriage is going well. Why would you want to risk toppling the balance by having a baby—or another baby?

More and more couples today are asking that question. Given that it is relatively expensive today to have a child, that virtually foolproof means of birth control are now available, that we have a new appreciation that not everyone is suited to be a parent, and most important, that women have a new selection of opportunities for careers outside the home, parenthood has become an option. We are members of the first generation to have the freedom of choice about parenthood, and we have the burden of decision that goes with that kind of freedom.

If you are now pondering parenthood, you are probably giving some attention to why you might want to, or not want to, have a child. If you are already pregnant, you probably also gave this question some thought and are likely to be still dealing with it, perhaps a bit perplexed at times about why you actually made such a momentous decision. What were you hoping to get—or give—from having a baby?

Your acceptance and understanding of why you decided to become a parent is a critical element in feeling comfortable about your status. Thus, before talking about the pregnancy experience itself, we will spend some time looking at the thoughts and motivations leading up to it.

Why are you going to—or why might you—have a baby? Before you can even begin to answer that question, you must accept the fact that the decision you make about having children is different from any other decision you have made or will make in the future.

By comparison, for instance, the decision to get married is an easier one to make. Before you say "I do" you've dated a number of people and have a good idea of the type of person you'd like to make a lifelong partner. And after you marry, you know that life won't really change drastically. Of course, there will be new ways of dividing up tasks, and adjustments you will have to make, but basically you will still be your own person. And, as you approach a decision on marriage, you have in the back of your mind an awareness that, if necessary, the decision can be reversed and the relationship dissolved.

The decision to have a child is different. The results are unpredictable. You have no idea what kind of person you will produce. You don't know how you will change or what life will be like if you do choose to be a parent. And, while you can have an ex-husband, ex-wife, or ex-job, you cannot have an ex-child. Parenthood decisions are irreversible and made without the benefit of relevant facts, and *that's* why they are unique.

Why do most couples have children? I've asked a few hundred couples that question over the past years and received in return dozens of blank stares, particularly from women who had a child or children ten or more years ago. "We never thought of *not* having children," a 50-year-old mother of three explained, referring to her own situation, but reflecting the views of the majority of men and women in her generation. "Actually, my whole life and upbringing was built around the assumption that I would have children some day," she continued. "My parents encouraged me to be a teacher solely because this would give me flexibility for family and career. It was assumed I'd have kids, and I never for a moment thought of not being a parent. So it just happened."

"I'm just old-fashioned enough to believe that children are the basic purpose of marriage," another woman in her sixties told me. "I simply don't understand all the discussion today about the 'whys' of having children. It's just done, that's all!"

A book published in 1939 had the promising title *Why Babies?*, suggesting that perhaps in earlier years there were some people interested in evaluating their motivation for parenthood. But it turns out that the subtitle of this book is *To Anyone with Any Sense It Should Be Perfectly Obvious Why*—and one of the chapters is entitled "Why to Have Four Babies."

A 1946 *Reader's Digest* piece (reprinted from *Cosmopolitan*) asked "What's Wrong with American Marriages?" and declared that what was wrong was that men and women were unrealistic and that "eager grooms and dreamy brides should realize that the true purpose of marriage is parenthood."

The fact is that until about 1970, parenthood was an expected part of married life and those married two or three years and not marching to the beat of bootied feet were pitied by friends and relatives. It was simply assumed that they were having difficulty becoming pregnant.

But today, instead of accepting parenthood as inevitable, more and more men and women feel that babies should be planned, arriving on a by-invitation-only basis. This abandonment of the "Don't think about it, just do it" philosophy is good in that it gives all of us a greater sense of control over the events in our lives, and increases the probability that children born today are very much wanted. Unfortunately, in our swing toward planning parenthood we may have gone too far, being overly critical of some of the very human feelings that tend to make having children attractive to us, posing the question of whether or not to have children on a solely rational, scientific basis while overlooking the highly emotional nature of that question. These overly rigid descriptions of "right" and "wrong" reasons may cause you guilt and anxiety during pregnancy and make you question whether your motivation was an acceptable, respectable, healthy one.

Why do people have children? In his book *Woman's Doctor,* Dr. William Sweeney writes that when he asks a woman why she is having a child, he waits for the response, "Because I like babies!" And various pieces of literature issued by Planned Parenthood state: "There are a lot of wrong reasons to have a child—but only one right reason—because you really want one." But what does "like babies" really mean, and how do you know what "really" is? And if you "want" one, *why* do you want one?

The Want Factor and Its Triggers

In saying, "I just want a child—that's my reason for having one," you are not revealing your actual motivation.

Something has to trigger your desire for pregnancy and parenthood. In addition to desiring a child for his or her own sake, if you are now pregnant or hoping to become pregnant, you are looking for something else as well. You see the possibility of a child as a way of fulfilling some current or future need. There is nothing wrong with that! *But as a first step toward making your pregnancy a successful psychological experience, you might try to identify the factors in your motivation.*

When parenthood began to be recognized as an option, a number of groups, including Planned Parenthood and the National Organization for Non-Parents, assembled lists of what they felt were the "wrong" reasons for having a child. Their intentions were good—they wanted to get people to think before they procreated—but, again, given that these or other groups have never issued a list of "good" reasons for parenthood, they may also cause some anxiety. Consider a few of the "dumb reasons" often cited, but this time from a different perspective. Perhaps in one or more of them you will begin to recognize some of your own motivations, and when and if you are challenged by someone about why you possibly might bring a new child into this already overcrowded world, you might offer a bit of personal insight of your own.

Babies and Marriage

"We're having a baby to save our marriage," admits an unhappy-looking couple on one of those lists of "reasons."

Surely you would agree that this is not an admirable reason to bring a new life into the world. Indeed, you might sarcastically comment that the only way a baby might help save an ailing marriage is by keeping the couple so busy they don't have time to fight. But under slightly different circumstances, this kind of motivation for parenthood perhaps is not so "dumb" after all.

"We have a feeling that a child will add more depth to our already strong relationship," was the way one husband I spoke with turned this reason into what was a "right" one for him and his wife.

"A child would be another person we could love and give attention to, adding a new type of richness to our already satisfying lives, creating an extension of ourselves, a living symbol of our love for each other," was how another woman described her and her husband's motivation for pregnancy.

Ellen, a 36-year-old public relations account executive, was still another person who felt that having a child would enhance her already good marriage, but her reasoning was a bit different from the two people mentioned above. "I always wanted to have a child—even more than I wanted to get married," she began. "For me it was finally finding the right man which triggered my immediate desire for a child. My father left our family when I was six. I saw the unhappiness it brought my mother and the havoc it wreaked with our lives. I never wanted that to happen to me. I've long wanted children, but only now with Bill does it seem right. I'm glad I waited. To me the concepts of wanting a child and having a good relationship in a marriage are inseparable."

Part of the rationale for warning couples to avoid seeking a pregnancy simply as an attempt to improve a relationship stems from the reality that babies can be a divisive factor. (Some cynics have suggested that the marriage vows be reworded to read "Until birth do us part.") But on the other side of that argument, they can offer some positive aspects, too. If you have seen the glow of mothers and fathers as they jointly embrace their sons and daughters, you understand those positive aspects. "My child is the 'we' of me," one young mother told me once. "You might even call her our own 'Mom and Pop art!' "

Families and the Future

"We're having a baby to take care of us when we're old," goes another of those "dumb" reasons for parenthood.

Now that really *is* a foolish reason, and you might want to warn people so motivated that instead of caring for you when you're old, children just help get you there faster. But on the other hand, you may want to admit to yourself that all of us have some anxiety—normal, healthy concerns—about the future, seeing a family base as a means of making that future a bit more secure, a little less unknown and frightening.

Ted, a 35-year-old banking executive, put it this way: "Julie and I never talk about children that much these days—she's only 25 and just getting started in her career. But I always get to thinking about having a family when I travel—especially on those long business trips across the country. Everything is fine when I get on the plane, but suddenly when I am 3,000 miles away, I begin to wonder who and where my family is. My parents are older, and a year or two from now it could be just Julie and me. I want more than that to come home to. It's funny how you have those thoughts when you're alone in a hotel room somewhere. But they are powerful and I can't put them out of my mind."

"I was always hesitant to have kids—my wife had to push me into it," a 40-year-old father of two and a successful architect confided to me. "But about a year after our first was born, my father died suddenly. It was really a shock. All I kept thinking was how lucky we were to have a son, that I still had a family and wasn't alone even though I had lost my father."

We do need others at every stage of our lives, and for many of us having a family can offer that feeling of security. Of course, you can't count on a child for either emotional or financial support. He or she may take off to Mars if transportation is available by then. On the other hand, as New York University School of Medicine psychiatrist Henry Greenbaum discussed with me, "Future security, however poorly defined that may be for an individual, can play an important role in the expression of desire to have a child. Man is the only species who knows about his death. He is aware of being mortal. We all have a fear of loneliness in old age, and we all worry about the possibility of being incapacitated. As life spans become even more prolonged, this aspect of family life may become even more important."

Critics of this motivation for parenthood are quick to point out that there are always friends, and that you should not create individuals just to provide an emotional cushion for yourselves. But generally the bond that exists between parent and child is unique. There *is* something different about a family relationship—the highs and lows, the daily problems, chuckles, hurts, needs, hopes—and for many couples contemplating parenthood, the desire for creating this type of close relationship consciously or unconsciously is an important part of their decision.

"I know it sounds funny—I'm almost embarrassed to mention it," a 32-year-old woman seeking help in making a decision about parenthood began hesitantly. She glanced at her husband and smiled, "But I began to wonder about who we would be spending the holidays with when we are sixty or seventy years old. Who would our family be? Do you think that is the wrong type of reason to want to have a child?"

That type of feeling cannot be labeled right or wrong out of context, but it can be categorized as a very common, although not always expressed, feeling of couples deciding to have a child. In a subtle way a child can provide a parent with a link with the future, a possible means of making the unknown a little bit less frightening. Demographically speaking, this may be particularly true for a woman. Since she lives an average of seven years longer than a man and is an average of three years younger than her husband, she has the possibility of ten lonely years to contemplate.

Often related to the feeling that children are a way of planning for the future is the desire in some way to perpetuate yourself, to leave some evidence that you lived on this earth. A 65-year-old man I spoke with expressed a rather dramatic example of this desire: "I was married for a very short time when I was in my early twenties. My wife and I had one child—a daughter whom I have seen only occasionally over the past few years. Recently my daughter had a child of her own—a little girl. When I saw the baby, I was suddenly overwhelmed with the realization that I had no one to carry on my name, that when I was gone, it would be like I never existed. I've had a mistress—a strictly business relationship until now. But recently I've invited her to move into my home. I want her to give me a son as soon as possible. It has become very important to me."

Is this a healthy approach to parenthood—the desire to have one's genes reproduced? Probably the way the above gentleman described his situation, no. But, on the other hand, a desire to recreate some of yourself in another human being may be a part, although perhaps a small part, of a whole configuration of motivations that predispose us toward wanting children.

Parenthood—"Something to Do"

"We're having a baby to give us something to do," a set of prospective parents on the "dumb reasons" list admits, as self-designated parenthood experts shake their fingers at them disapprovingly.

But again, there are other ways of viewing this motivation toward parenthood.

Terry, a 29-year-old physician who became pregnant while she was in a residency program in psychiatry, explained, "I'm not exactly looking for something to do. I work twelve hours a day, have only a few days off each month, have to keep house and keep a husband happy, too. But I began to wonder recently if I might not like to have something *different* to do, something that would be new and refreshing. I know that having a child will mean I'll have less time for the professional work from which I derive so much satisfaction. But in return I'll be gaining a whole new vantage point on life, experiencing emotions, activities, pains, and pleasures which I would not otherwise know."

" 'So what?' I asked myself," she continued. "If I see 500 fewer patients, or write 100 fewer professional papers in the next 25 years, would I or the world suffer a great loss? I really don't think so. But perhaps I would suffer a great loss by filling my life with only work-related matters. You know, I don't think I have what you'd call a maternal heart. I don't really like other people's children. But I know I'll love mine."

Having a child just because you have nothing else to do is hardly an admirable type of motivation. But it is viewed by many as a basic life experience. "I think that most couples in their twenties and thirties who are thinking ahead to possibly becoming parents want to know what the experience of parenting will be like for them," states Dr. Amy Miller-Cohen, who with her husband, Dr. Robert D. Cohen, runs a New York–based parenthood counseling service called Pondering Parenthood. "They may have had little experience, together or separately, being with babies and children, and they are curious about themselves as caregivers, as well as about babies and children. These are exciting, uncharted territories. For older couples there is also heightened curiosity about the biological, reproductive capabilities. Men may be waiting to know if they are really fertile and a woman's capacity to bear a child may have been unused for so long that she is strongly motivated to find out if she can reproduce and what it will be like."

To acknowledge the female desire to experience the physiological (as well as postbirth) events related to pregnancy is not necessarily the same as concluding that there is some biological drive toward motherhood. Rather, it emphasizes that pregnancy and childbirth are uniquely female functions about which most women are curious and generally inclined to want to experience at least once.

(There are those who claim that there *is* some biological urge involved here. Simone de Beauvoir, in *The Second Sex*, writes: "It is in maternity that woman fulfills her physiological destiny; it is her natural 'calling' since her whole organic structure is adapted for the perpetuation of the species." And Dr. Helene Deutsch, in *The Psychology of Women*, states that pregnancy is "the direct fulfillment of the deepest and most powerful wish of a woman.")

Is "wanting something to do" a common motivation for parenthood? "Yes—but that's a funny way of putting it," a 25-year-old woman reflected, as her husband, two years older, looked on and nodded in agreement. "It's more a matter of wanting something special and very meaningful to do, and in the process, hopefully benefitting yourself. I had my children because I simply wanted to have the thrill of seeing them grow and develop. And I thought that they would help us grow, too." Her husband spoke up: "There were times when we didn't have kids that we began to feel that we were too much in our private world, out of touch with some of the more basic human problems that surround us, perhaps a bit lacking in compassion for others who are more dependent, more helpless than we are. Basically, we saw parenthood as an opportunity to grow ourselves, to focus on problems and challenges other than those directly affecting us."

Children can give you something to do. They can provide a challenge through which we test ourselves. We can grow through them, learn the basics of life all over again. As Goethe wrote, "You have to ask children and birds how cherries and strawberries taste."

"Reasons" for Having Children: A Perspective

In the midst of all the discussions about planning parenthood and thinking through the parenthood decision before acting upon it, many couples—perhaps you among them—began to assume that there was some totally sacred, selfless reason to have a child. And they became confused as a result, often feeling guilty and self-critical about some very basic human feelings. In evaluating your own motivations toward parenthood, remember that children are not asking to be born. In deciding to have children, we are attempting to meet some current or future need. We have babies, if we do, for emotional, self-serving reasons.

Once you've acknowledged this and accepted the fact that the scientific method has limited use in weighing motivations for parenthood, you are well on your way to feeling comfortable with whatever decision you make.

Whatever individual or series of motivations—some of what may be what Angela Barron McBride in her book *The Growth and Development of Mothers* called the "normal crazy reasons"—triggered or will trigger your own desire to have a child, they are by definition "good reasons" and are sure to stay off any list of "dumb reasons" if you have what we might call the "Want Factor," *a sincere desire to welcome a child into your life and the readiness to share your time, love, and attention with a new human being.* Your decision to have a child is "right" if you are ready to accept what Simone de Beauvoir called "a solemn obligation."

Is There a Best Time to Have a Child?

If you *are* going to have a child, is there any time that will be better than others to have him or her? Is there a time that will be convenient in terms of juggling parenthood and a joint career? How late can you postpone childbearing and still hope for a problem-free pregnancy? How do you know when you are emotionally ready to accept the responsibilities that go with raising a new human being? In short, when is the best time for you to have a first or later baby?

Right now, if you've already made the decision and are expecting a child—whether it is the right time or not!—these questions may seem a bit too late for you. But some brief comments here may serve to allay some fears you now have, and suggest ways that you can deal with problems should they occur. If you are still contemplating the "when" of parenthood, this discussion should be right on target.

Marriage Stability

Dan and Alice didn't rush into marriage. They dated for the four years of college, were engaged at the beginning of their senior year and married just after graduation. Their future together looked bright. But within months after their wedding, as they began to experience life off the campus, their relationship took a turn for the worse.

Alice, a high school English teacher, works fairly regular hours and has a considerable amount of free time in the evenings after preparing for the next day's classes. It did not take her long to develop a deep resentment for Dan's late hours at the office and his frequent business trips. She frequently complained of being left alone, ignored, isolated. The more she complained, the more deeply Dan seemed to become involved in his work, and the wider the gap between them grew.

In her moments of isolation and depression, Alice considered what she thought could be an effective solution to their problem: "If we had a baby, I think things would be different," she explained. "Maybe then Dan would have more interest in home life. And I'd have something to do. I think a child could give us more of a life together."

One might legitimately question Alice's motivation for parenthood at this time. As we've already discussed, having a child to fill in a gap in one's own life, possibly to patch up a deteriorating marriage, is hardly an admirable motivation for creating a baby. Parenthood can offer a new dimension, a new type of richness to a marital relationship, but it certainly cannot make up for shortcomings that existed beforehand. Indeed, the reality is that the first child brings many psychological changes to marriage, producing a negative impact within people who are highly immature, secretly dependent, and themselves wish to be children. For Alice, motherhood might complicate her domestic problems. At a time when her primary attention should be on resolving her differences with Dan, she'd be giving her full time and attention to a new child.

Given the current high divorce rate, it is neither pessimistic nor impractical to assess your marriage, making sure it is well grounded before deciding to turn a twosome into a threesome. Certainly every couple has some problems, some source of conflict; however, a significant disagreement or general lack of communication may well be reason enough to postpone parenthood.

Having a baby very soon after you are married, even if the child is conceived after the wedding, may not be ideal, because most marriages take some time to "settle down." Yet it can be argued that there is such a thing as waiting *too* long after marriage to have a baby. You may get too used to having things your way, too accustomed to being just the two of you, and the transition to parenthood may be more difficult to make.

Self-Knowledge, Self-Confidence

Kathy, aged 28, felt considerable pressure in making the decision about when to become a mother. "I don't want to wait until it's too late. Everyone tells me that I should have a baby right now. After all, we've been married seven years and we're very happy together."

"I know we want a child—at least one," she continued. "But somehow something is wrong about having one right now. I haven't quite figured myself out yet. I've been working as an executive secretary ever since I got out of college, but I really want to do more. I've been thinking about getting a masters degree in business, or some other type of specialized training. My fear is that if I *do* have a child now, I'll be locked in. I haven't done what *I* want to do yet. I might resent the child for holding me back, competing with me for my time . . ."

Obviously, you can't count on postponing parenthood until you've achieved what you believe to be complete success in your career. First, that time may never come, and second, if it ever does, you may be past the reproductive years. But you can get yourself established, get a feeling that you know your own nook in life. A marriage should be a combination of two complete individuals, not a man and a woman who are looking to each other for mutual completion, and the approach to parenthood should be the same. Prospective parents should try to establish their own identity before they participate in creating a new, separate one. Most important, you should guard against creating a child as a means of filling an otherwise empty life.

The benefits of postponing parenthood until you really know yourself and where you are going in life are multifold: You'll feel more comfortable with your decision to have a baby; you'll be likely to welcome the child more enthusiastically, with fewer reservations, fewer second thoughts; you'll have more to offer a newborn child if you, yourself, are a complete person.

Long-Term Plans

"I don't want to be too old to enjoy life with my kids," Walter, a 28-year-old medical intern told me. "When they are teenagers I don't want to be old and grey. I figure if we start our family now I'll be in my forties by the time they start college and I'll be in my fifties when they have my grandchildren. I know some parents who I feel waited too long—and were so old they couldn't relate to their children at various stages of their lives."

This "generation factor" may or may not be important in determining your family planning scheme, but, again, it is something you may want to consider, at least briefly.

Similarly, your final family size—and the timing of second and later children—might also be significant in planning the birth of your first. If you are now 27, are planning to have three children at three- or four-year intervals, and want to complete your childbearing by the mid- to late thirties, then, all other things being equal, you'd probably want to start now. On the other hand, if at age 27 you want to have two children, closely spaced, you may feel you have more flexibility.

Timing the Logistics

There may be no completely convenient time to be pregnant and care for a newborn infant but, on the other hand, if you really do want a child, there are times which are less inconvenient than others. The key to handling the practical questions is being both realistic and flexible.

Take your career plans into account. You may not want to miss a great opportunity in your chosen profession or feel that you have to take a leave of absence before you are at least somewhat established. Were you to do so, you might harbor some resentment which would interfere with the development of the intimate emotional relationship you'll want to develop with your child. By assessing the current and future situation at your office, you may be able to find a logical time for "intermission." But on the other hand, you should attempt to avoid being unrealistic in your evaluation. Ask yourself if your job will really be less demanding a year or two from now, if you will be traveling less, having a more regular work schedule. "I have been saying for the past two years that my job was just too hectic right now to take time to have a baby," one 39-year-old advertising executive told me, "but all of a sudden I realized that my job was *always* going to be hectic. So now is as good—or as bad—a time as any to take off some time."

Being realistic here will help you avoid postponements which may result in your having a child when it is actually less, rather than more, convenient. Similarly, if it is finances that concern you, do some calculations to predict, to the extent that you can, what your future economic situation will be. Yes, it is expensive to have a child, and it is nice to have some money put aside before starting a family. But if you do some careful thinking and predicting, you may find that, given the inflation that is likely to be with us for the next few years, the difference between right now and three years from now in terms of how much money you have available might not be all that significant.

In coping with practicalities, be flexible. Don't lock yourself into thinking there is just one way of doing things. For example, having a baby doesn't mean that you have to leave your apartment and move to a house, or to a larger house. There are ways of managing, either by getting larger living quarters or doing some clever rearranging in the place you have. And becoming a mother doesn't automatically mean that you have to sever all ties with the business world. Of course, life will change if you have a baby. If you are currently working nine or ten hours a day at an office job, something will have to give if the child is to get the attention he or she deserves. But there are ways of working out part-time assignments, or taking a limited leave of absence during the first few months or year of a child's life.

Making The Decision

Very few childfree couples escape proparenthood pressure. And even fewer parents with one child manage to avoid the "helpful" advice of relatives and friends who want to know, "When are you going to give little Johnny (or Mary) a brother (or sister)?" Additionally, there is the advice of those who may tell you that you should enjoy being childfree as long as possible, maybe forever, noting that having children may be a real drag compared to pursuing an exciting career outside the home.

Even if you and your husband are left alone to decide about the if and when of parenthood, the thought process can be complex. Ideally, both of you should be in agreement about that "if and when." In reality, it doesn't always work that way. "We both are very positive about having a family," Molly, a 30-year-old actress, told me, "but my husband wants to wait another four or five years. He says he will be ready then. But I'm ready now, and I just think it would be foolish to postpone having a child just because he has a vague feeling that he needs more time."

In some cases, of course, the man is not only hesitant about having a baby when his wife suggests, but is hesitant about having one at all, perhaps even adamantly against it. "We talked about having children before we were married," Emily, a 33-year-old scientist expecting her first child, told me. She looked a bit depressed as she spoke. "Every time I raised the subject he would say, 'Someday, later, maybe.' I finally realized that this postponement could go on so long that we might never have children. And I knew I wanted at least one. Finally, I had to confront the issue head-on and say, 'Look, I don't want to wait any longer.' And I did conceive. But I would hardly say he was a willing participant in the whole process.

I'm hoping that he will come around as the pregnancy progresses."

Perhaps it is because a woman is more vividly aware of the biological limits on her childbearing potential, but whatever the reason, it is more common for her to bring up the topic of the "when" of having a baby. Very often a man *is* hesitant. Often he *does* need to be nudged some. Indeed, after speaking to dozens of couples about this specific issue I have concluded that if we all waited to have our husbands sing the glories of parenthood before we conceived, children would be on the list of endangered species.

Of course it can work the other way too—the husband being eager to start a family, the wife stalling for more time. "I'm a grammar school teacher," a young father declared, "and I simply love kids. I think I saw having a child as a means of consummating our marriage, making it really forever. And I wanted one right away. But my wife had other things to do with her life, so she kept me on a string for a while."

"My husband is the born-father type," another expectant mother explained, "and has been for years asking me, 'Are you ready now?' Well, until recently I wasn't ready. Why? Because, quite honestly, I didn't want to compete with a child. I was so lacking in self-confidence that I thought he would prefer the child to me. Only when I began to feel better about myself did I come to the point where I could say, 'I'm ready.'"

What we are talking about here is differences of opinion between husband and wife on the issue of *when* to have children, not more serious conflicts about whether or not to have them at all. Obviously, if the conflict about the question of parenthood is more fundamental than simply the timing of it, you might want to seek outside professional help, either through a carefully chosen preparenthood counseling specialist, marriage counselor, psychiatrist, or psychologist.

The decision of whether or not to have a child is a highly personal one, influenced by individually determined emotional and practical factors. But a few general guidelines might help resolve any quandaries or conflicts you have.

First, don't let pressures influence your decision. Relatives and friends who are "concerned" that you are not reproducing on schedule can be given polite explanations of your feelings of uncertainty about parenthood, or less polite reminders that it is none of their business.

Second, sort out real concerns from smoke screens. Career and life-style factors and doubts about parenting ability may be authentic concerns, or they may be cover-ups for more serious qualms about having children, ranging anywhere from hostility toward a spouse or a miserable childhood experience of one's own to a possible fear of childbirth. It may help to spell out the pros and cons in writing, or free-associate into a tape recorder. Ask yourself if you'd still be undecided if your life circumstances were very different, say if you suddenly became very wealthy. By doing so, you may be able to separate deep psychological conflicts ("I do not like children" or "I am too insecure in my marriage to invite children") from logistical problems ("We can't afford a baby right now" . . . "Having a child would require us to move to larger quarters" . . . "There is no way I could keep my job and have a baby too").

Third, if logistics are a concern, make a realistic evaluation. Study your professional and social calendar for the past two weeks and think about what modifications would have to be made if you had a child. Be honest about how you feel about rearranging or modifying your lifestyle. Don't expect miraculous new forms of cooperation from a husband who has always left everything to you.

Fourth, think "person," not baby. The concept of "baby" may discourage couples who envision parenthood as an endless sequence of bottles and diapers; or it may encourage people taken by the image of an angelic cherub, but horrified by the continuous responsibility for someone who will be an infant, a toddler, a school-age child, and a young adult.

Making up your mind about having a baby would be much easier if you could expect that one day a bell will ring, a smile will come to your face, and you would then know for sure you had the answer. But don't hold out for that day: it won't come. If you really know yourself, it can't come, because by relying on such an extreme you'd be denying the very ambivalences and conflicts that characterize us as human.

It's fine to plan, to talk about parenthood, to go through all the pros and cons of having a child. But after digesting all the facts, doing elaborate cost/benefit analyses, going through a myriad of other intellectual exercises, you must realize you're dealing with an emotional decision. Perhaps for the first time in our life, you will have to admit to yourself that you can't have all the answers—you simply do not know what the future will bring. In deciding to have a child, you are taking a leap of faith.

Seeking a Pregnancy: What's Your Style?

With all this discussion about deciding to have children, it must be acknowledged that there are a number of different ways the conception of babies occurs.

First, despite the fact that we live in the Age of The Pill, some babies are the result of old-fashioned bungles of love. "I was using the diaphragm, but it just didn't work. And I know the exact night it didn't work," claimed one new mother, speaking somewhat defensively. Well, maybe. But the chances are these "accidental pregnancies" may involve more than mechanical failure on the part of the birth control method.

Second, there are those who approach parenthood very romantically, as exemplified in this woman's experience: "My husband came home one night three months ago, put his arms around me and started getting very amorous as I was making dinner. 'Let's start a baby tonight,' he said. I was a bit surprised—but also very excited, because I had been waiting for a year for him to come around to my way of thinking on that subject. We made love that night, and although I doubt that was the exact time our baby was conceived, we will always remember it as the night we began our first child."

Third, there are those who take the "let's see what happens" approach. They make a very subtle decision to let pregnancy occur. "We didn't really try to conceive," an expectant mother in her midtwenties explained. "We just stopped using birth control. I really can't recall any particular day when we turned to each other and said, 'Let's give it a try.' We talked about having and wanting children, joked about the day I stopped taking The Pill. But that's about as close to a formal decision as we came."

Linda Matthews, one of the authors of *The Balancing Act: A Career and a Baby,* was in this "let's see" category: "For the first time in my life I couldn't get myself to use the diaphragm . . . then I was pregnant. Both of us realized that it had been no accident, but a confirmation of our relationship."

Fourth, there is the "plan everything out" type of couple who enters parenthood with a calendar, thermometer, and a great deal of enthusiasm. "I figured that once we finally decided 'yes,' that we might as well not waste any time," a woman in her third month told me. "I took my temperature for two months to get an idea of what was going on, and then the next month we had sex at just the right time. I got pregnant right away."

"We talked about having a baby for four years. All of a sudden both of us became very enthusiastic about the idea—and we couldn't wait to begin one," another woman related as her husband laughed, recalling the circumstances. "We decided one night we wanted a baby as soon as possible, and I was so annoyed that it was the wrong time biologically. I can tell when I'm ovulating, so the next month, the morning I felt it, I told my husband. He called into work saying he was sick, went out and got a couple of bottles of wine, lots of cheese, and we spent the whole day in bed making our baby!" Her husband picked up the conversation. "We wanted the conception of our child to be special—we wanted to remember the event. There is a scene in Harold Pinter's play *The Homecoming* in which the son confronts his father, asking him to describe the circumstances of his conception—he really wanted to know the background of how he came into existence. Now we can tell our child."

While a day off in bed with wine and cheese may appeal to you, the possibility of making pregnancy a scientific expedition probably does not. Couples who have difficulty conceiving often have no choice but to plan their love life around a calendar and thermometer (one woman told me that two dinner guests who were an hour late arrived breathless, explaining their lateness because the wife's temperature had suddenly risen as they were about to leave), but unless you have to, you will probably want to let your pregnancy occur more spontaneously. ("This trying-to-get-pregnant bit sure can take all the sex out of intercourse," is how one man who very much wanted to be a father put it.)

Whatever the circumstances and whatever "trying" technique you choose, you may well begin to feel differently about sex—and about each other—as soon as you omit birth control and realize that pregnancy is a possibility. "We felt positively giddy after sex," one woman declared. "We kept thinking, 'Well, tonight may have been the night.'" She shook her head and laughed nervously. "Of course, that all changed after we didn't conceive right away. Then we just plain worried."

In an ideal world, you should be enthusiastically bubbling with joy about having the baby you are seeking, both when you are "trying" and when you find out you are pregnant. But true confessions are in order. "Even as we were trying to get pregnant I wondered if I was doing the right thing," a high school teacher who was then four months pregnant confessed. "I kept thinking about how drastically a child would change my life. And as the time for my period approached, I couldn't figure out if I wanted to get it or hoped it wouldn't appear."

The subject of ambivalence is very much part of the whole pregnancy experience, and begins to manifest itself even before conception. It occurs because you are dealing with an unknown, and you cannot know at this point if the decision you made is in your spouse's—best interest. You will not be able to rid yourself of these second, nagging thoughts. You can only learn to live with them, not be defeated by them, and avoid having them spoil what otherwise would be a psychologically successful pregnancy experience.

THE PHYSICAL

Preparing Your Body for Pregnancy

Much of the fear and anxiety you may experience during your pregnancy can stem from concerns that you did not do everything "right" from the very start, that you may have done something, or omitted something, which will adversely affect the child.

So, "before the fact," set the stage for a healthy pregnancy by taking advantage of these five tips.

First, have your physician evaluate your rubella, or "German measles" status. Rubella is a common, mild, infectious disease of childhood. For many years it was assumed to be an atypical form of measles or scarlet fever. But in the early 1940s it was discovered that, unlike either of these two other diseases, exposure to rubella during the first three months of pregnancy can have devastating effects on the developing child. Cell division is somehow inhibited and the child may be born with such congenital defects as deafness, cardiac malformation, and/or cataracts. Be sure you are immune to rubella!

The chances are over 80 percent that you already are. You were most likely exposed to the disease during childhood. It's highly infectious, yet also very mild, so you may not have ever known you had it. Ask for a rubella screening test. It may take a couple of weeks to get the results, so plan accordingly. Do not try to conceive or let conception occur until you get the results. If you do not have rubella antibodies in your system, or if there is some doubt, you should get the vaccination as soon as possible, and postpone conception for at least three months after the immunization (which actually gives you a mild case of the disease).

Second, take a critical look at your current use of tobacco, alcohol, and drugs. Chapter 2 describes in detail some of the hazards of these three categories of substances,[1] but right now what is important is your commitment to giving up all forms of tobacco and drugs

---

1. If you now smoke, drink, or use drugs regularly and are contemplating pregnancy, or are now pregnant, read pages 72–74 immediately.

(unless a drug is specifically recommended by a physician who knows you are seeking pregnancy), and either abstaining from alcohol or using it in moderation (no more than one, occasionally two, drinks containing one ounce of liquor a day). This advice is particularly important for the would-be mother, but is also relevant to the father because drug, alcohol, and tobacco use may—among other things—influence his ability to impregnate.

Third, if you are using the oral contraceptive as your means of birth control, give yourself two or three months without The Pill, choosing some other form of contraceptive; for example, a diaphragm or condom. This break from The Pill will give your body a chance to return to its normal menstrual cycle, making the calculation of your due date somewhat easier, and will eliminate the possibility of Pill-related pregnancy problems which occur infrequently, but are nevertheless worthy of attention.

Fourth, make sure you are eating properly. In the months before you conceive, you need a normal, varied, balanced, moderate diet. To insure this, choose a number of foods from the Basic Four food groups (milk and dairy products; meat, fish, and poultry; cereals and breads; and fruits and vegetables), making sure you have two moderate servings from each category every day. Check your calorie needs with a standard height-weight-age chart and keep within the recommended range.

Obviously, the months before pregnancy are definitely not the time to try one of the many fad diets that are now circulating (actually, no time is!). You should be building up your store of nutrients in preparation for the all-important early weeks of pregnancy. You will not, for example, be doing yourself—or your future child—justice by eliminating carbohydrates from your diet in an effort to have the "fat burn off."

Fifth, plan to have a prepregnancy physical examination to review your general health status. Tell your physician of your plans to have a child and raise at that time any questions that are on your mind. For example, if you have a family history of any hereditary disease— such as diabetes, sickle cell anemia, cystic fibrosis—you may want to discuss with him the possibility of genetic counseling.

This discussion of physical preparenthood planning may initially seem irrelevant to our general discussion of pregnancy as a psychological experience. But if pregnancy does occur while you are, for example, still smoking cigarettes, drinking heavily, using some form of drugs, or generally worried that you are not in good physical shape, the nagging anxiety that you will have to deal with for nine months can be emotionally devastating. As we'll discuss in the next chapter, for a number of couples the anxieties that they "did something wrong" at or about the time of conception spoiled what could otherwise have been a very special, very happy occasion: the day they learned they were expecting a baby.

How Long Will It Take?

There are some interesting psychological characteristics among couples who are "trying" to get pregnant.

Many are very secretive about their decision, perhaps not even verbally acknowledging to each other that they are "trying" for fear of building up expectations that perhaps won't be met. More likely than not, the "trying" couple does not announce their intentions to the world. By doing so they would only be surrounding themselves with unnecessary pressure. "I told my office-mate that John and I hope to have a baby soon," one 30-year-old magazine editor admitted to me. "And now I wish I'd kept that fact to myself. We've been trying for five months and nothing has happened, and every once in a while, I get the feeling she looks at me, thinking 'Well?' "

For many couples the subject of whether or not they are able to have children is a very sensitive one. After all, you never do know until you try. "My husband and I waited six years before we had our first child," one mother, now expecting her second, explained. "We got all the normal teasing about not having kids. But then one day my aunt announced at a family dinner party that she thought it was so sad that we were sterile. I was furious! I never realized until that moment how sensitive I was on the subject. While we were trying to conceive it was very much on my mind—I mean, wondering if my aunt was right."

"I am very anxious about the whole topic," a 35-year-old author informed me. "I had an abortion nine years ago and I must admit that ever since then I have wondered if I ever would be able to conceive again. My husband wonders too. We've only been trying two months, but both times when my period arrived we were both in the dumps for a day or two."

"It was a very stressful time for us," related one mother who bounced her two-month-old son on her lap while she talked. "My husband and I were both in college when I first conceived, and he felt we just couldn't have the child. Against my will, I had an abortion. I never have been able to forget that—and, in a way, I held it against him. If I wasn't able to conceive after that I probably couldn't have forgiven him. So while we were trying, we both were very tense."

When you seek a pregnancy, your ego is on the line. If you now harbor some fears about your ability to conceive or impregnate, consider yourself normal. Don't make things worse by setting unrealistic goals for yourself; specifically, don't expect to conceive the first month you try. Don't panic if pregnancy does not occur exactly on the schedule you have devised. Considering that a woman's egg is available for fertilization only some 12–24 hours a month, and that a sperm may be able to live and retain its ability to do what it does best only during the 48 hours before ovulation, you're talking about a period of 72 hours per month during which sex may lead to pregnancy.[2]

If you have sexual relations five times during the month, the probability of conception occurring in the first month is about 16 percent. Obviously, you can increase these odds by having inter-

---

2. There is some disagreement about the length of the fertile period; it may be longer than 48 hours, possibly 96 hours in length.

Some couples today are interested in the timing and length of the fertile period for reasons of influencing the odds on the sex of their offspring. Scientific studies now indicate that early-cycle insemination resulting from sexual intercourse, as opposed to artificial insemination, will increase your odds of having a male child. Intercourse at the time of ovulation will increase your odds of having a female child. These conclusions (detailed in my book *Boy or Girl?: The Sex Selection Technique That Makes All Others Obsolete*) are just the opposite of those offered by Dr. Landrum Shettles and others in the late 1960s. The apparent discrepancy is explained by the fact that early investigations in this area were limited to cases of artificial insemination and it was assumed, inaccurately, that the conclusions would apply to natural insemination.

course more frequently, especially during the most fertile portions of the cycle—that is, the day before your temperature rises.[3]

You'll still hear, "Oh, we decided on Monday we wanted a baby and on Tuesday I was pregnant." But in the great majority of cases it just doesn't work that way. So in planning your pregnancy experience, be flexible. Don't work out a strict timetable for yourself once you decide "yes" and stop using contraception. Just relax and see what happens.

3. If you have a regular cycle, the day before the temperature rises is the one occurring 14 or 15 days *before* the beginning of your next menstrual period. In a 28-day cycle, this would mean that the most fertile days would be days 13 and 14. If your cycle is longer than 28 days, the fertile period would be later; if the cycle is shorter, the fertile period would be earlier. If you are having difficulty identifying your fertile period, the temperature charts in *Boy or Girl?* may be helpful to you.

CHAPTER 2

Just a Little Bit Pregnant

(Months 1 and 2)

THE PSYCHOLOGICAL

Finding Out

Susan, a junior high school chemistry teacher, and Art, both in their late twenties now, had postponed parenthood until a time when they felt they were settled in their jobs and had put aside enough money to live well on just his income. I met with them in the living room of their home, an old house they had purchased a few years before and were redecorating room by room. Both described themselves as "simply loving kids." With shoulder-length, straight blond hair, Susan's tall slim figure hardly revealed that she was four months pregnant. Art, a high school football coach with dark hair and a muscular build, had an arm around his wife as we talked.

"It didn't happen the way we planned," Susan began, laughing nervously as she related their story. "I was the type who would run home at noon if I had forgotten my pill. I was terrified of having a baby before we were ready to take care of him or her." She sighed and went on. "Finally, the time seemed right. I stopped The Pill—and that next month I was sure I was pregnant. I remember complaining to Art about how fast it had happened, wondering if we didn't need more time. And then I went trooping off to the doctor, only to have him tell me I wasn't pregnant. I burst into tears, realizing for the first time how much I did want a baby—and right away.

"We tried for months after that. And nothing happened." She shook her head bitterly, then spoke with more emphasis. "And let me tell you, I was incredibly depressed every time I read about all the women who wanted abortions or when I would see a pregnant teenager in my class. Here I so much wanted a child and I couldn't have one!"

Art picked up the conversation. "We started making the rounds of the infertility specialists in town, but they couldn't find much—except that Susan wasn't ovulating as regularly as she should. Basically, they said 'Relax.' But how could we? We wanted a baby so much! No joke, we could actually paper a few large rooms with all the temperature charts we have. Those schedules don't do too much for your sex life. I began to feel like a trained seal. And every month it would be the same. She'd get her period and we'd both be depressed for days, and then it would start all over again."

Susan smiled, but a bit sadly at the recollection. "Each month I lived in hope that I was pregnant, and every time I was a few days late my mind was racing with thoughts of motherhood. Finally, one of the doctors I was seeing decided I should try a new type of fertility drug. After 18 months of disappointment, I was ready to try anything! Before I started on the drugs he gave me a physical and then told me to call in for another appointment so he could start me on the fertility medicine. She paused, gulped audibly, and went on. "So between classes one Friday—I'll never forget the day—I called his nurse for an appointment. She was very coy and said, 'Hold on for a second, Mrs. James.' The doctor came on the line and said, 'Guess who doesn't need fertility pills! Congratulations, you're going to be a mother!' " Susan had tears in her eyes as she described her reaction to the news. "I managed to contain myself for about thirty seconds until I got into the ladies room, then I just cried and cried with happiness. A miracle had happened. It was just the biggest birthday cake in the world!"

"How did you learn the good news?" I asked Art. He seemed pleased to have the opportunity to talk about what was obviously a very special occasion for him.

"Susan told me later that she had rushed home from school to prepare a very special dinner. She wanted candlelight and the works when she told me. But it didn't work that way. She couldn't keep the news to herself for one minute. When I walked through the door she threw herself into my arms, crying, 'I'm pregnant, I'm pregnant!'

"Of course I was thrilled—but I have to tell you more honestly, I was stunned. Although we'd been trying for months, prospective fatherhood was the furthest thing from my mind at that moment. I was really caught off guard. I couldn't believe it." He looked at Susan and laughed. "I kept saying, 'Are you sure? Are you sure?' We sat down on the couch and didn't say very much, just feeling very grateful, very happy, very close to each other."

"Was your reaction uniformly positive?" I addressed the question to both of them. Susan spoke first.

"At first, yes. All I could think of was that I had at last achieved a very special goal, one which I had been striving for for months. I was absolutely elated, on top of the world. But later on that night, I came down—just a little bit. I thought, 'My God, this means my life is ending, that another life is beginning!' I began to face the reality of having a baby, how it meant I had to leave my job, how expenses would mount up. We had forgotten about all those down-to-earth things during our months of trying and hoping. And then they started to come back to me."

"To me, too," Art added. "I got our bank account out that night, and started to do some calculating, like how we were going to meet the mortgage payments without Susan's income. But I wasn't worried enough to let it spoil our happiness."

Anna (three months pregnant at the time I talked with her) and Fred were 32 and 35, respectively, and had been married for seven years before their first child was conceived. She was an attorney who worked with a small midtown law firm. Fred, who was not present when I met with her at a cafe near her office, was a business executive in a downtown insurance company.

"We talked a great deal about having children before we were married," she began. "I think Fred was concerned that with my career in law and my commitment to working, I wouldn't want kids." She laughed in a way that expressed more than a bit of irony. "I assured him I did and there were ways of successfully handling both. But neither of us wanted children right away—we thought we needed at least two years to ourselves." She paused, looking very thoughtfully at the floor, and went on. "Well, those first two years came and went and there was no talk of a child. We were both so busy—both at work and socially—and we travelled a lot too. So the subject didn't come up that much. Finally, about two years ago, I said, 'Why don't we think about having a baby?' and was, frankly, surprised and very hurt that he was not enthusiastic.

"Something must have happened in those five years to convince him that children were a burden—and a thankless one at that, because that's what he stressed in our conversations. I kept after him, but he was still as down as ever about the idea. We love each other so much and are so happy together, the fact that we didn't see eye to

eye about a child didn't—and still doesn't—make any sense to me.
Then one night a few months ago I got into bed and told him, 'I'm
not using the diaphragm this time.' He didn't say very much. And
that was that.

"My periods aren't terribly regular anyway, so the fact that I was
late that month didn't really surprise me. Again, I was pretty busy
and put the subject out of my mind. Then, when I was two weeks
overdue—and that's late, even for me—I was walking down the
street and a girl handed me one of those little booklets advertising a
free pregnancy test. Obviously, it was an abortion center seeking
clients. But I decided to take them up on their offer." She laughed,
"I was really new at all of this! I called them and they told me to
bring a morning urine sample in a sterilized bottle. Heaven only
knows why it had to be sterilized! Well, I hadn't the slightest idea
where to get such a container—so I went to the drugstore and
bought a baby's nursing bottle and boiled it. That seemed appropriate at the time! I took the sample in and the receptionist told me to
call her the next morning at 10 for the results.

"I never mentioned anything to Fred. Quite frankly, I was afraid
to. The next morning at work I started to call the pregnancy center.
But each time I simply couldn't finish dialing. I don't know what I
was afraid of—finding out I was pregnant or finding out I wasn't. Finally, at 4:00 I mustered up enough courage to call and get the
news." Anna took a gulp of coffee before she continued. "I think that
was the longest minute of my life—I mean, when the woman at the
office said, 'Hold on, I'll check.' Then she simply told me it was positive and asked if I wanted to come in for 'counselling.' I declined
and hung up. And I stared into space. I guess you could say I was
both excited and terrified. I remember I left work early and wan-
dered aimlessly through a park we have near our apartment. I'd
never seen so many babies in that park before! My main problem at
that point was how to tell Fred. Then I got an idea. On the way
home I bought three large jars of pickles and put them side by side
in the front of the refrigerator. He always makes himself a drink
when he gets home—and knows that neither of us eats pickles that
often.

"Well, he came home, opened the refrigerator and then came out
to the living room, looking as if he'd just seen a ghost. He simply

asked, 'Is it true?' I nodded. He stood still for a moment, then went into the den and closed the door, staying there for what seemed like an hour." Anna shrugged her shoulders and shook her head. "Let's say that is not exactly the type of reaction I had thought I'd have when I told my husband we were expecting a child. I was so hurt, I went into the bedroom and sobbed." She stopped for a moment to collect her thoughts and regain her composure. "Finally he came out and put his arms around me and said something like, 'It will work out okay.' But he was so distant and he still is. I guess I have enough confidence in our relationship to know that by the time the baby is born he will have adjusted to the idea. And I know he will be a good father. But right now, it is incredibly difficult for me. You know, I have second thoughts myself about having a baby—with my job and all. I need someone to give me some emotional support and confidence. I feel very alone right now."

Jill, a 24-year-old interior decorator, and Peter, 25, who owns and runs a small furniture store, were expecting their first child in five months when we met on the terrace of their one-bedroom apartment. They told me right away that they had planned to start a family two years after they were married and, keeping to their schedule, they stopped using birth control on the eve of their second anniversary.

"We both knew, obviously, that pregnancy was a possibility," Jill, a petite brunette with a rosy complexion and an almost constant smile, told me, "but we didn't want to make a big deal about trying. If it happened, fine. And it did happen much faster than we thought!" She laughed, patting her slightly enlarged abdomen. "Two weeks after we stopped using birth control, I was having lunch with a client and had this overwhelming urge to have a glass of milk. I *never* drink milk! Then a few days after that, it was Thanksgiving and we went to Peter's family's home. As usual, my father-in-law offered me a cocktail. I'm hardly what you'd call a big drinker, but I don't turn down one or two, or maybe three on a special occasion. But this time I simply didn't feel like having it. Then I knew for sure something was going on."

"I began to suspect, too," Peter said. "The night after Thanksgiving I was making one of my special fish casseroles, something she usually likes, but this time the smell revolted her. She went into the bedroom to take 'a little nap' at 6:30 and woke up fully dressed at 7 the next morning."

Jill smiled and picked up the conversation. "We really didn't talk about the subject directly—but I think we both kind of knew. Finally, I thought I should have one of those bunny tests and I asked Peter to take the urine sample into the lab near his office. That afternoon, while I was working at home, they called me with the news.

"How did I react? I can only say that I was stunned and elated. And I was absolutely *dying* to tell someone. But I didn't want to call Peter at the office. I wanted to tell him in person. And I was afraid it was a bit too early to tell our parents or friends." She thought for a moment and went on, searching her memory for details of that day. "I remember going out late in the afternoon to buy a pair of boots. My usual size was a big snug and I explained to the saleslady, 'Well, that's normal; you see, I'm pregnant.' She was *very* enthusiastic. And I felt very good having told someone!"

Peter had something to say. "I had no idea how long it took to get test results—I thought at least a few days. So it wasn't on my mind when we met at a little—and very informal—restaurant near our house. I got there before she did. I saw her walk in dressed in this brand new, long, ultra-suede skirt I had gotten her for her birthday a few weeks before. 'Why in the world are you wearing that here?' I asked. And that's when she told me, 'Well, dear, it seems that I won't be fitting into it too much longer.' " He sat back in his chair, looked at Jill and laughed. She picked up, "He was very, very quiet when he got the news. As I remember, he ate less than half his dinner that night."

"Were you pleased that you were expecting a child?"

Jill answered first. "I guess on a scale of 1 to 10, with 10 being overjoyed, I was about 7. I'd say the critical point is that we didn't expect it to happen so fast. We weren't really trying! And there it was. I have found out there is a big difference between talking about the possibility of becoming pregnant and actually finding yourself in that condition. As soon as I began to suspect that I could be, my whole attitude about life changed. I began thinking of working more at home, rescheduling our vacation so we would relax before I got so big that we couldn't travel easily. I began to project ahead about this new life I had inside me, wondering what he would be like—and I did think from the beginning that it would be a 'he.' I still have a few of my high school biology texts in the bookshelf. I got them out— and all of a sudden those very scientific-looking pictures took on a real meaning. 'My baby looks like that,' I thought. I developed an instant distaste for that very cold term 'fetus.' It was always a baby to me." Jill bit her lip thoughtfully, then continued.

"I'll tell you, there were a few things that really did worry me—I mean, in addition to the normal things, like could we afford it, and where would we put it. As we told you, we didn't really think I'd get pregnant so fast. And I had promised myself that I'd give up smo- king—I mean the marijuana, too—beforehand. So when I found out I was pregnant and remembered that around that time we had got- ten pretty high on a few weekends, I did worry. Like how could I have been so stupid? My doctor said it was probably nothing to tor- ture myself about because I'm not a heavy user, but I wish now I hadn't smoked at all.

"And I had a few other worries right after I learned that I was pregnant. I somehow kept thinking that maybe it was all a mistake, that maybe I would get my period and the test was wrong. I just didn't feel all that different—no morning sickness or anything. So I kept looking for some confirmation that something was really in there. Oh, and another thing—something that really surprised me. Right after I got the call from the lab, I started to get a little bit anx- ious about labor and delivery. My mother really had laid a heavy trip on me about that subject—you know, 'Listen to what I went through for you.' I hadn't really thought about it for years, but some of those fears suddenly resurfaced. I had a dream about a week later that I was carried out of the delivery room in a casket. I'm pretty much over that now. I've read enough to know it just couldn't be that bad. But that worry was there for a while."

"Do you want to know what concerned me most?" Peter asked. Then he sat back and put his chin in his hand. "I felt a bit left out —right away. I mean she was pregnant. And who was I? Where did I fit into all of this? I will candidly admit that I felt a bit jealous. Someone else was going to come into our lives, and that might mean less of Jill's time for me. For the first week or so she seemed so quiet, so very involved with herself."

Reaction: Mixed

As these three couples exemplify, there can be a full gamut of reactions to the news of a pregnancy. Certainly your life circumstances are important in determining that reaction—an unmarried 18-year-old couple is bound to react differently than would a long-married 30-year-old couple. And men and women who have long tried to have a very much wanted baby and finally succeed will be more positive, indeed joyous, in their reaction [1] than the couple for whom pregnancy, while planned, happened sooner than expected. Additionally, the manner in which you find out can influence your immediate response. If you gradually begin to drift into an awareness that conception has occurred, perhaps feeling that you "just knew" right from the start, the circumstances may be different than if your doctor, in the course of a routine examination, says bluntly, "You're pregnant."

Reactions can be different, but upon hearing that you are going to be a mother or father, it is very likely that you will feel some ambivalence. Your feelings probably will not be 100 percent positive or 100 percent negative.

On the positive side, you are likely to have at least a passing flash of pride over the fact that you could do it—that is, become pregnant or impregnate. "It confirmed my identity as a woman—both for myself and for people around me," a young advertising executive and mother of two sons told me. "I had the feeling that many of my relatives thought that I could be a success at business, but would never succeed as a woman. The moment I found I was pregnant I felt like a more complete person. And it gave me great pleasure to tell some of my relatives who, I felt, thought I would never make it."

---

1. *Reader's Digest* a number of years ago carried the story about a couple who had long tried to have a child. Finally they sought medical help. The physician in question called the husband one afternoon at work with his bad news: the wife had a physical problem which meant that she could never conceive. The husband was understandably distraught and delayed going home that night, trying to figure out how to break the news to his wife. When he finally walked through the door his wife was distraught "Where have you been?" she asked "I've been waiting for you for hours—I've got wonderful news! I'm pregnant!"

The sheer wonder of finding out that a new human life has been created is likely to add a sense of excitement and wonder to your contemplation of the news.

As Jill mentioned, pictures of babies developing in the womb can suddenly fascinate you. Oriana Fallaci, in *Letters to a Child Never Born*, begins a dialogue with the fetus even before the pregnancy test is confirmed ("Last night I knew you existed," she says to this developing person she calls "Child"), and she covers her bedroom walls with the scientific pictures of the occupant of her womb. (She continues: "I've cut out the photograph that shows you at exactly two months; a closeup of your face enlarged 40 times. I've pinned it to the wall and lying here in bed I'm admiring it: haunted by your eyes . . . what do they see? You won't raise your eyelids again until the sixth month. For twenty weeks you'll live in complete darkness. What a pity! Or is it?")

You may have a surge of protective feelings toward this new life, a warm sense of attachment even at this early stage. A number of women who, after learning of their pregnancy immediately made an appointment for an abortion, have told me that even they wanted to nurture this fetus ("I drank a quart of milk a day") although it was not to survive. Additionally, your initial reaction may be colored by positive thoughts of what your future may now bring, the hope that this new child offers in terms of an enriched, fuller life. You may be pleased at the prospect of telling others your good news, especially those who you know have long anticipated the event and are bound to share your happiness.

But on the other hand, your reaction will probably not be all positive. "Although I was thrilled, I was also apprehensive at the same time," Joan, a 30-year-old high school teacher, told me. "There was just so much else going on in our lives right then. I had just started a new job, we had just moved into a new house and had months of redecorating ahead of us. I began to question whether this was really the most convenient time. And I got downright scared about the responsibility I had suddenly assumed. How did I know we could handle it? It seemed a bit late at that point to be asking questions, but I did anyway. Did I really want this baby? I always thought I wanted one, but now I'm not sure."

A wide variety of unusual circumstances can color your reaction.

"I prayed for a pregnancy for years," one mother told me. "Finally we gave up on having one of our own and we adopted our son Billy. We absolutely adore him, and have done everything to ensure that we treat him as though he were our biological child. Then to everyone's surprise, I got pregnant. What would otherwise have been a reaction of excitement and joy was marred by my fear that we would possibly act or feel differently toward our two children, no matter how we tried."

The stereotype of a woman learning she is pregnant is one of total joy and contentment. There has been much discussion about the enigmatic smile of Mona Lisa, observers long having commented that she is smiling because she has just learned she is pregnant. Interestingly, however, the *New England Journal of Medicine* once carried a letter from a reader that suggested, "To one unencumbered by the sophistication of the obstetricians and historians, that smug, sly smile can have only one explanation: Mona Lisa just discovered she is *not* pregnant." Probably the smile could be suitable for both occasions, depending on the circumstances.

Ambivalence after you learn of your pregnancy may manifest itself in many ways. You may shiver and want to run the other way when you pass the maternity or baby clothes department in a store. You may be looking for signs that your period is indeed going to come, dreading it and hoping for it at the same time. You may experience transient periods of deep depression. Studies have shown that early in pregnancy, as many as half of women who enthusiastically planned the conception have serious second thoughts after the fact. And the percentage of those with marked ambivalence is likely to be much higher among those whose pregnancy "just happened."

Telling Him

In a modern-day book on pregnancy, you might not think there is a need for a section about breaking the news to your husband.

After all, pregnancies are more likely to be planned, husbands more likely to be aware of the possibility of pregnancy and its signs, couples more likely to speak openly about the subject. While it is true that most women no longer feel they have to break the news by furiously knitting baby clothes or by fainting in the parlor, the news is usually not received simultaneously by both expectant parents.

First, when seeking a pregnancy, some couples are sensitive enough about the subject that they don't discuss it with each other after The Decision to Try is made. It usually *is* a very emotionally charged issue. Perhaps they are afraid to raise false hopes or set themselves up for failure.

Second, given that even in our age of presumed equality and sameness, biological differences still remain, it is usually the woman who finds out "for sure" first and that sets a situation for "telling him."

For years, you may have imagined what it would be like to tell your husband that you are pregnant for the first time. The typically anticipated sequence of events you had in mind probably was this: subtle hint, direct announcement, gasp of joy, enthusiastic embrace, and within minutes, the sound of a popping champagne cork. But sometimes it just doesn't happen that way. The reaction instead may be a dropped jaw, a glazed stare, utter speechlessness, and two scotches—both for him.

Any reaction is possible. "I called Bill at the office the moment I got the news. And he yelled 'WHOOPEE' so loud that everyone in his office heard him," one expectant mother told me. "He called practically everyone he knew that night. We had no secret to keep!"

"I let my husband know by phone, too," her companion added. "He was so excited that we went out to celebrate with the boys and didn't come home until after midnight."

Sometimes the expression of joy is more subtle, more emotionally based. "It was a very special night for us," a very pregnant nursing student holding her husband's hand explained, relaying what has to be every woman's expectation of the ideal circumstances. "He came home from work, plopped down on the couch. I sat in his lap and said, 'Do you love me ? Do you love me enough to have a baby with me?' We just embraced for a long time. We were both overwhelmed with emotion. We were very happy in our own quiet way. And ever since then he kisses me twice every night, once for me and once for the baby."

Sometimes the reaction appears to be neutral, neither very positive nor very negative. "I can only describe my reaction as stunned," a new father recollected. "It was a Saturday and she got a call from the lab. She hit me with an enthusiastic, 'Guess what! And I kept saying, "Are you sure? Are you sure?' "

The circumstances under which the pregnancy occurred are bound to determine his reaction, much the way the circumstances colored your initial view. Anna and Fred's situation (where his reaction was less than enthusiastic) is not at all unusual. "I was heartsick for days after I told him," another young mother of two confided to me. "We had planned to have children someday. But I guess my 'someday' came before his. I had to push him into the decision. And when I told him he was simply depressed. He told me he wasn't sure he wanted to have a child, not sure he was cut out to be a father. I didn't know how to interpret what he was saying. Was he really saying he didn't want me to be the mother of his children? In the past I always criticized him for not expressing his feelings to me. But on this occasion, I wish he had kept his feelings to himself."

Sometimes the reaction of a husband who has agreed half-heartedly to "try" to seek a pregnancy is even more negative. "I really dreaded telling my husband," a 35-year-old mother of a year-old daughter told me. "We never discussed having children before we were married. He has three kids by a previous marriage and was not eager to start all over again. But as I got older, I decided I really wanted one. We discussed it—actually, we fought about it a lot. Finally he stopped resisting and I didn't use the diaphragm for a few months. When I told him I was pregnant he sat down, put his head in his hands and said, 'I was playing Russian roulette and I lost.' Evidently he was hoping and praying that I wouldn't conceive. He was very low during the whole pregnancy. He's cheered up considerably ever since. But I still get the message he feels that he did one very big favor for me, one which he hopes to cash in on some day."

Some men—as some women—are quite depressed, very glum, withdrawn, when they receive the news of pregnancy. In the situation above, where the man had the financial responsibilities for two families, one can see a practical reason for his concern, although by acknowledging that, we are not condoning his lack of emotional support. But other negative reactions may be a bit more difficult to understand. Perhaps it could be that he is once removed from the immediate events. While in the back of his mind he might have been aware that pregnancy that month was a possibility, he was probably not focusing on it in the same way you were; he was not looking for signs and symptoms that would suggest your efforts had been successful. While you've been through the motions involved in getting a pregnancy test and awaiting the news, the announcement to him comes out of context. He may be pondering the day's stock market results when you inform him he is to be a father. He's caught a bit off guard, without the immediate emotional preparation you've had when you got the news.

"I got the news while I was on a business trip," a distinguished corporate executive recalled. "I phoned in from a telephone booth at the airport—every time I'm in that airport I vividly remember that booth. She told me; I said, 'Congratulations.' But I was really unprepared. I was on the road for another three days and did a lot of thinking. I needed that time. By the time I got home I was tremendously excited about the baby."

His first reaction, if it is not all positive, may reflect a number of conflicting feelings. It might reflect some jealousy (as Peter explained) over losing his exclusive relationship with you. Or there can be Peter's feeling of "Where do I fit into this?" The fact is that jokes are made about expectant fathers, that they are often ignored in discussions of pregnancy. (It has been said that the only books that focus any significant amount of attention on fathers are Blackstone's law books.)

Or, his first reaction may reflect a feeling of loss of control over the events in his life. "I felt that suddenly this enormously important event had happened, and there was no going back to my old life, whether I wanted to or not," was the way one expectant father explained it, adding, "There is only one way of describing it—I was scared, frightened to death." His reactions may include a component of "What, now? . . . Us?—parents?" ("I always assumed I'd be a father. But always later, not now. When 'someday' became 'now,' I was stunned. Having children is what other people did, not us.")

Or the immediate thought may be of the enormous economic burden he is assuming for at least 18 years. "My attitude toward my job changed instantly," one new father told me. "I stopped speculating in the market. And I began keeping a budget. I had never been responsible for anyone before in my life. I felt the burden immediately."

As the proverb goes, "A father is a banker provided by nature," and as the old joke goes, "The tenth month of pregnancy is worse for the father, because then he is carrying the child." Very often the initial response of a man, particularly a relatively young one, when he learns of the pregnancy, is one of tremendous insecurity about his ability to provide, or resentment that he has been strapped with what he feels is a financial burden.

And his reaction may even reflect a little bit of a very normal sense of doubt. Is it his child? How can he be sure? As a French proverb states, "Maternity is a matter of fact, but paternity is a matter of opinion."

What is the solution to the problem of an unenthusiastic expectant father? Before even attempting to offer a solution, one point should be made clear. Unless a woman has deliberately sought to deceive her husband, planning without his knowledge a pregnancy that he definitely did not want, it is really unforgivable for a man to abandon his wife emotionally at this crucial time. The majority of women who experienced this lack of support told me it evoked a feeling of aloneness and despair that they might never be able to fully forget.

One mother of two offered her ideas on the subject. "I was hurt that he didn't jump for joy when I told him. But I made an effort to get him involved from the beginning, showing him pictures of what our baby looked like at four, six, eight weeks. He is such an enthusiastic father now, it's hard for me to believe that I worried back then over his coolness. Maybe there should be a society for previously hesitant, but now delighted, new fathers who could offer counsel to expectant parents, help allay their fears and anxieties."

Dr. E. E. Masters, director of and professor at the School of Social Work at the University of Wisconsin, states that "Parenthood (not marriage) marks the final transition to maturity and adult responsibility in our culture. Thus the arrival of the first child forces young married couples to take the last painful step into the adult world." Sometimes this step represents a type of life crisis for both a man and a woman, and their relationship together.

Secret or General Announcement?

Some couples want to tell everyone their news as soon as they themselves know. "I didn't even wait for the test," an editor of a scientific journal told me. "The morning my temperature was up for the sixteenth day I called my mother and said, "I think I'm pregnant."

"When we were engaged we didn't tell a soul," another new mother recalled, "and that was no fun at all. I don't like keeping my joy to myself. So when we found out a baby was coming we told all our friends right away."

But there is at least an equal chance that you, for one reason or another, will want to keep your pregnancy your own secret for the first few weeks. The most commonly offered reason for the great conspiracy is fear of miscarriage. "I knew my parents would be absolutely delighted to hear that, at last, they were going to have a grandchild. But I wanted to get beyond the first weeks, to make sure I was going to really stay pregnant," was the way one woman put it, reflecting the views of many others. "I could hardly believe myself that I was really pregnant, so I figured I ought to get used to the idea myself before I told others," was another common reaction.

"I used to write the Class Notes for my college magazine," a woman in her ninth month told me, "and we were always told never to announce pregnancies, only births. In my early months I began to understand why there was such a rule. Since most miscarriages occur in the first 10 weeks, I wanted to get out of the danger zone before I made my news known. To do otherwise seemed to be setting myself up for the possibility of tragedy."

You may enjoy your secret, smiling mysteriously at those noticeably pregnant women you pass on the street. Or you may be frustrated by it. ("I kept hoping someone, like my mother, would say, 'Gee, you look different. Why?' Then I would be forced to tell.")

THE PHYSICAL

If your pregnancy is well planned, perhaps even using a thermometer to detect your most fertile time, you will probably be very aware during the days after conception that pregnancy has possibly occurred. If you are taking your temperature, you have a "natural pregnancy test" available by simply continuing to take it for the two weeks after ovulation: If your temperature remains elevated for 16 days and you are not ill or have any other explanation for the higher temperature, the overwhelming odds are that you are pregnant.[2]

If you're not taking your temperature and begin to suspect you're pregnant, the first thing you are likely to do is get a urine or blood type of pregnancy test. All of these tests look for the presence of the hormone HCG (Human Chorionic Gonadotropin) which is secreted by the early version of the placenta and is present in most concentrated form in the first morning urine. The tests usually can detect a positive reading about three weeks after conception has occured; that is, about one week or 10 days after your period is due. But most laboratories ask you to wait until you are at least two weeks "late," preferably a little longer, before you submit a urine sample. Depending on the type of test used, you will be given results in five minutes to 24 hours. ("Bunnies" are too expensive these days; most labs now use biological materials rather than animals of any variety.)

Although the tests are 95 percent accurate, only a physical examination will confirm pregnancy. By the time you are six to ten weeks pregnant the inspection of your cervix will show that it is slightly bluish in color and that your uterus is now slightly enlarged. By that time, of course, you will probably be aware of your breasts enlarging and feeling more tender than usual, with the nipple and surrounding colored area (the areola) darkening somewhat; you might also

2. If, from temperature charts, you know the date of the insemination which led to pregnancy, you can calculate your approximate due date by adding 266 days to that date. If you don't know when conception occurred, the due date is assumed to be 280 days after the date of the first day of your last menstrual period. This latter method is generally an accurate means of estimating, except for women who tend to have long menstrual cycles—31 days or more. In that case, the 280-day method probably results in a due date that is five to ten days earlier than birth is likely to occur.

notice increased urination, an overwhelming desire to fall asleep in the middle of the day, and possibly some slight nausea.

When you are "a little bit pregnant" dramatic changes are occurring throughout your body. As early as 20 days after conception, the baby's backbone, nervous system, and spinal canal are being formed. The foundation for the child's brain has been established and a primitive heart begins to beat. By the seventh week (counting from the first day of your last menstrual period) the chest and abdomen are completely formed, eyes are clearly perceptible through closed lids, the jaw is now well formed, lung buds have appeared, the big toes are visible and, although you are unaware of it, the fetus may begin to move his or her body ever so slightly. By the eighth week, the face and features are established, as are the teeth and facial muscles. By the ninth week the legs, hands, and feet are partially grown, and the fetus is beginning to look like a miniature infant, being about as large as the first segment of your thumb.

In the course of all this internal growth, there are often some anxieties and some external symptoms that cause concern. At this stage of your pregnancy certain things should *not* concern you, at least not to the extent that they make pregnancy unpleasant. But certain other factors are of great importance and merit both your concern and attention.

Don't *Be Concerned About* . . .

Nausea

Some 60 percent of women experience nausea of some kind during the first two or three months of pregnancy. The physiological reason for it is clear: your digestive processes are slowed down during early pregnancy, and due to a decreased production of acid in the stomach, the food just sits there, producing a sensation of fullness. It may be a worrisome discomfort to you. ("I was fine all day, but every night around dinnertime I began to feel awful. It really interfered with what my husband considered the most peaceful time of our day—alone, together. I just couldn't come to the table for a few weeks.") Or it may be a reassuring sign. ("Although the test was positive, I never really believed it until I began to feel nauseous in the morning. This sounds a bit foolish, but it was comforting. When I felt queasy I would say to myself, 'See, you really are pregnant.' ")

Psychoanalaysts have offered elaborate explanations for the nausea and vomiting of early pregnancy, telling us that there is a constant struggle in pregnant women, both to preserve and destruct the fetus, and that vomiting represents an unconscious attempt to expel the fetus. Nonsense. It is a temporary physical reaction which you can deal with by eating small amounts of food frequently, instead of forcing three large meals on yourself; alternating solid and liquid foods at the same meals; avoiding rich, greasy menus that are hard to digest even in a nonpregnant state; and nibbling on crackers or lightly buttered toast. If nausea is not controlled in this manner, tell your physician and he may prescribe some perfectly harmless antinausea medication.

Sex Hurting the Baby

Unless your doctor specifically tells you that sex during the first months after conception poses a risk—and explains to you why it does—you should not be concerned about continuing your normal sex life, if, of course, you feel like doing so. There is no biological basis for the widely recommended rule of avoiding intercourse on those days when you would normally be expecting your period. Indeed it is difficult to uncover exactly what piece of medical information ever led to that "rule" in the first place. Similarly, there is no basis for concern about intercourse early in pregnancy introducing "germs" or other sources of infection. The embryo, soon to become a fetus, is well protected right from the start.[3]

You may find that your sex life improves in the early months of pregnancy. "It was terrific!" one expectant father exclaimed. "We had tried for months to conceive and sex was getting to be a real

3. It should be noted that many of the books written in the early part of this century for the pregnant woman assumed or recommended that "marital relations" were inadvisable. One published in 1916, *The Diary of an Expectant Mother*, told of how the husband immediately began sleeping in the living room as soon as the pregnancy was confirmed.

drag. Now we can make love whenever we want to, not when the thermometer and calendar tell us we have to."

"It was all of the fun and none of the responsibility," another soon-to-be father told me, his wife adding, "Being pregnant contributed a new dimension to our already loving relationship. It was marvelous."

On the other hand, you may find that you are not very interested in sex in the early months of pregnancy. Masters and Johnson, in their various studies of sexual response, reported a decreased interest in the first three months of pregnancy, although Elisabeth Bing and Libby Colman, in their excellent book *Making Love During Pregnancy*, report no low point at this time. You may find you are simply too tired at the end of the day (try some other times!) or that you feel too nauseous for any activity whatsoever. Your sexual pattern and frequency will be your own, but unless otherwise advised by your physician, set aside your fears about sexual intercourse and orgasm being a threat to the fetus.

Psychic Influences

In 1881 a medical journal reported the case of one Mrs. Wilkins who had an uncontrollable desire for oysters, but couldn't find them to eat. She and her doctor were terribly worried that this great desire would mark the child, and the journal offered a solution: Tell the woman to put her hands on her buttocks and pray fervently that if the marks must occur, they would be at that location. Later the editors proudly reported that the baby was born with a large mark in the form of an oyster on his rear end.

For years both before and after that date, women have been told by friends, relatives, and even some physicians, that their state of mind could influence the child—that they should be spared excitement, not see a fire, not be bitten by a dog or have a tooth pulled. This is good old-fashioned hogwash, perhaps somewhat entertaining, but nonetheless hogwash. Keep it off your list of concerns. Certainly a greatly disturbed mental or emotional condition can have physical ramifications which could harm the child, but everyday events—including brief episodes of grief, fright, or anxiety—are not important in terms of the child's development.

Miscarriage

The overwhelming percentage of miscarriages occur so early that the new cells have not yet implanted in the uterus, and neither the woman nor her physician is aware that pregnancy has occurred. But the possibility of miscarriage you are concerned about is the type that might happen, however infrequently, in a later part of the first three months. This is one of the many aspects of pregnancy which is out of your control, so there is no constructive purpose to be accomplished by worrying about it. You can, however, be aware of symptoms of impending miscarriage.

If one is in the offing, the bleeding is likely to start as a dark red or brown staining. Over the course of four or five days, it increases to an amount larger than a normal menstrual period and becomes bright red. Medical treatment is available for heading off a threatened miscarriage, but when it cannot be prevented, it is most often interpreted as a lost opportunity rather than a lost baby—and the couple is eager to start a new pregnancy as soon as possible. Very often an early miscarriage is the direct result of a cellular defect in either the egg or sperm, or an imperfection in either conception or implantation. It is very rarely the result of something you have done, and thus if it does happen, nothing to berate yourself or feel guilty about. Once you have completed 10 or 12 weeks of pregnancy, counting from the first day of your last menstrual period, you can be confident that the time of major risk of miscarriage has passed.

Abnormalities

"Will my baby be normal?" Probably no expectant parent ever escapes that worry at some point. During the first two months this concern will probably manifest itself (and probably intensify later before it begins to fade in importance). While we'll have more to say about this concern later, right now you should be able to handle this anxiety by studying the statistics: About 1 in every 200 to 250 pregnancies is affected by a chromosomal abnormality of some type; 88 percent of those pregnancies end naturally, usually in the first few weeks after the missed menstrual period. If you have no family history of any inherited disease, the odds are overwhelmingly in favor of a successful pregnancy and delivery of a healthy baby.

Rh Factor

At least right *now*, don't be concerned about it. Your Rh status really has nothing to do with conception or early pregnancy, but it can be significant at childbirth. For that reason, your blood must be tested for the presence or absence of the Rh factor, now generally a routine procedure.

Some 86 percent of the population have Rh positive blood; the remainder have Rh negative blood, which is not at all compatible with the positive variety. If your blood is Rh negative, your husband's blood will also be tested. If he, too, is Rh negative, or lacks certain of the Rh subfactors, in all likelihood your baby will also be Rh negative and there will be no problem. If, however, your husband is Rh positive, there is a good chance your baby will also carry the Rh factor.

During the process of delivery, a small amount of fetal blood may be released into your bloodstream. If you are Rh negative and your baby Rh positive—and *if* any mixing of blood should occur at birth—your body will immediately begin producing antibodies against this "foreign" substance, much as it would against a bacterial invader. This presents no problem for your firstborn child—and possibly not for your second, or even later children. But should your body have built up these anti-Rh antibodies to any great extent they *could* affect a subsequent baby by reacting against its red blood cells and causing the condition known as erythroblastosis fetalis—or what is sometimes referred to as an "Rh baby." A simple blood test performed on the baby immediately after birth, and repeated during the early weeks of life, assures prompt detection and treatment.

None of this, however, need be any real source of concern today since a drug treatment administered to the mother right after birth can prevent formation of the Rh antibodies, thus virtually eliminating the complication just discussed. But it *is* important that your doctor know ahead of time if you are Rh negative.

Be *Concerned About . . .*

Getting the Medical Care That's Right for You

You should see a physician or other type of health professional specializing in the care of pregnant women as soon as you suspect you are pregnant. Very rarely something does go wrong early in pregnancy (for example, an ectopic pregnancy, where the fertilized cell settles somewhere other than in the uterus, most often in the Fallopian tube).

Begin to think about what type of relationship you want with the person who will be overseeing your health during this important eight-month period (assuming you seek help when you are one month pregnant). Is it important to you to have someone you can talk with, confide in, someone who is not so brusque in his or her approach that you get two clinical minutes of time at each visit, and that's it? (If you're paying top dollar, you *should* expect, indeed demand, a significant amount of attention.) Is affiliation with a certain hospital important to you? Will you consider having your prenatal care handled by a certified nurse-midwife instead of a physician? Is price an important part of your decision? (In the New York City area, at least, obstetrician fees generally range between $1,000 and $2,000, confirming the observation that OBs, like storks, can have big bills.)

An increasing number of women, although still a minority, after considering these questions, are turning to the services of certified nurse-midwives. Barbara Brennan (herself a certified nurse-midwife) and Joan Rattner Heilman discuss this option in detail in their book *The Complete Book of Midwifery*, describing the large-scale midwifery effort which has been in process at the Roosevelt Hospital in New York City since 1974. They note that the midwife used to be a "granny," an untrained birthing assistant, but is now a specialist with obstetric nursing experience and graduate training in midwifery. All but three states (Michigan, Massachusetts, Wisconsin) now permit nurse-midwives to practice, and the costs involved, as compared to a physician's fees, are significantly lower. (At the Roosevelt program the all-inclusive fee for prenatal care, postpartum visits, delivery, and a 48-hour hospital stay, is $899, and is cov-

ered by many insurance programs.) Any complications, such as a
Caesarean section or the use of forceps, involves the assistance of a
physician and extra fees.

There really are no guidelines for the best way to choose a doctor
or midwife. Make a list of the characteristics and other points that
are important to you, and do some shopping around. Contact
friends who have recently been pregnant and discuss their experiences. Don't do what one woman did, choosing a doctor on the basis
of one, inflexible criterion: "All I wanted was a doctor who could
promise both painless childbirth, and that if the baby was abnormal
at birth he wouldn't let it live. I ended up choosing a man who was
cold and totally disinterested in my case. When it came time to
deliver, he wasn't even there, and an intern had to help deliver my
baby."

Drugs

For centuries it was thought that the placenta acts as a barrier,
protecting the fetus from all but the most severe assaults by outside
sources. We now know that the protective capacity of the placenta is
limited.

If you take certain drugs during your pregnancy, they may result
in abnormalities in the fetus. This lesson was brought home all too
dramatically by the thalidomide tragedy. Don't take any drug without consulting your doctor, and that includes over-the-counter
drugs, too. If you have taken some form of medication at about the
time you became pregnant, tell your physician about it. ("I was taking sleeping pills right around the time I conceived," a woman in
her sixth month of pregnancy told me, "and I worried about it for
four months before I had the nerve to ask my doctor. He checked
out the drug and told me I had nothing to worry about.")

In addition to avoiding drugs which are not approved by your
doctor, be cautious about the use of X-rays. The amount of radiation
exposure in a diagnostic X-ray is extremely small and consequently
results in an infinitesimal increase in the rate of genetic change.
From a practical point of view, there is nothing to be concerned
about from one, or even a few, diagnostic X-rays during pregnancy,
if they are medically necessary. But caution is advised. Tell any

physician or dentist you visit that you are pregnant and, if possible, postpone the X-ray until after your baby is born.

Cigarette Smoking

As with drug use, smoking is a cause for very real concern during pregnancy. Both epidemiological and experimental studies unanimously support the view that smoking has a retarding effect on fetal growth. Analyses of hundreds of thousands of births have shown that the average birth weight of babies born to smoking mothers is a full 6.1 ounces less than those born to mothers who didn't smoke. Also, significantly more babies under five pounds are born to women who smoke, and their pregnancies last for a shorter time. Recently, the *New England Journal of Medicine* added a new item on the already long list of cigarette-induced tragedies: Women who smoke are at least twice as likely to suffer a miscarriage as women who do not smoke.

The problems associated with low birth weight are well documented. These babies are often disadvantaged from the moment of birth through the early years of their lives, perhaps longer. A large study conducted in England concluded that "the mortality in babies of smokers was significantly higher than that of nonsmokers." The same study raised questions about the long-term effect of smoking during pregnancy on those babies who do survive: Children of smokers followed up during their early years were found to be significantly shorter, to have low ratings of "social adjustment," and greater frequency of reading retardation. It's not smart to smoke anytime, but during pregnancy, it's really unforgivable.

And it's not just the mother-to-be who should kick the habit. The prospective father should too. The effect of exhaled cigarette smoke on a fetus has not yet been fully measured, but there is reason to believe that it, too, could be harmful. Besides, after the child is born you'll be particularly conscious of the adverse effect exhaled smoke can have on growing children, particularly with regard to development of respiratory problems.[4]

4. If you feel you need help in giving up cigarettes, call your local chapter of the American Cancer Society. They will provide you with literature and can recommend some professional groups, including the local branch of the national organization Smoke-Enders.

Alcohol

A substantial number of children born to women who drink excessively while pregnant have a pattern of physical and mental birth defects referred to as the "fetal alcohol syndrome." Growth deficiency is one of the most prominent symptoms. Affected babies are abnormally small at birth, especially in head size. Unlike many small newborns, these youngsters never catch up to normal growth. Fetal alcohol syndrome babies usually have narrow eyes and low nasal bridges with short upturned noses. Almost half have heart defects, which in some cases require heart surgery.

What should you decide about alcohol use during pregnancy? You might want to consider abstaining completely from all forms of alcohol, especially in the first three months of your pregnancy, when the most fundamental structural fetal development takes place. (You might have this problem solved for you if cocktails all of a sudden lose their previous appeal, perhaps tasting very bitter. One woman reported that she always enjoyed a couple of glasses of white wine with dinner, but couldn't tolerate the taste until her fourth month—and then only with a teaspoon of sugar mixed into the glass to make the beverage go down.)

But if you choose not to abstain, drink moderately, perhaps a glass of wine a day, or occasionally one or two ounces of 80-proof liquor a day. Stay *well below* that limit during the first three months. Women have consumed alcohol during pregnancy for years, and we have no reason to believe that small amounts will prove harmful. But large amounts of alcohol and pregnancy definitely do not mix well.

Nutrition

Although it may come as a surprise to you, in your early months of pregnancy you don't need anything but a normal, well-balanced diet. Your caloric needs are not increased—yet. Get your 2100 calories (or whatever is advised for your nonpregnant height and weight) by having two to four glasses of skim milk; two servings of meat, chicken, or fish; one egg; four servings of fruits and vegetables (including citrus and dark green, leafy, or yellow vegetables); four servings of bread or cereal.

Although your doctor will probably offer you vitamin supplements, you should be aware that this is more likely to be an "insurance policy" rather than a necessity. The National Research Council recently looked into the desirability of vitamin supplements in pregnancy and concluded that they were generally of "questionable value," the exceptions being iron and possibly the B vitamin folic acid, both of which are difficult to get in sufficient amounts from a normal diet. You'll want to take your own doctor's advice on the subject of supplements and feel comfortable with the knowledge that while they may not help a great deal if you are eating properly, they won't hurt you or the baby. Beware of self-prescribing your own "megavitamins." Those *can* be hazardous to your health and to your baby's health.[5]

We'll look more closely at the "food psychology of pregnancy" in the next chapter, but suffice it to say here that right now is a good time to muster up all the motivation you possibly can to avoid the "well-I'm-pregnant-so-I-should-indulge-myself" pitfall that many women fall into. Pregnancy is a time when you want to pamper yourself and have other people show you special considerations. But those considerations should not include extra rich desserts and two helpings of everything that precedes dessert.

Drugs, cigarette smoking, excessive use of alcohol, and diet—those are things which you have reason to be concerned about. Those are areas in which you can take positive action to protect your unborn child's health. But don't delude yourself by thinking that all of these are necessarily of equal importance. For example, don't assume that it's permissible to smoke because you are being very careful about your diet, assuming the nutritional effort will compensate for the cigarettes. It won't. Indeed, while diet during pregnancy is important, much more harm can be done to your baby by smoking cigarettes or drinking large amounts of alcohol. During World War II in parts of Europe, rationing led to a situation where expectant mothers were allowed only 800 calories a day—and prob-

5. In addition to not needing megavitamins, you do not need any so-called health foods. There is no reason that you need avoid artificially flavored or colored foods, or products artificially sweetened with saccharin. Moderation here, as with all food products, is the key.

ably not very nutritionally balanced calories at that. The babies born to them were normal, although in many cases a bit smaller than usual. On the other hand, repeated scientific studies have shown that tobacco and excessive drinking can cause very, very serious problems.

Smoking, drinking heavily, using unapproved drugs, eating poorly, are in themselves harmful to the baby. But they can psychologically hurt you too—perhaps for many years to come. The example of a depressed and very guilt-ridden 32-year-old new mother is appropriate here: "My son was born six weeks early. He weighed four pounds. I ate right, didn't drink much, never went near even one aspirin, but I couldn't give up the cigarettes. Not that I enjoyed them, but I couldn't quit. I would light up and the whole time worry, thinking of the poster showing the pregnant woman smoking and her child coughing violently inside her. But I still smoked. When I went into labor so early, I knew why—it had to be the cigarettes. And when I saw how small he was . . ." She stopped abruptly, then went on. "I'm not sure my husband will ever forgive me. I torture myself thinking about it. Every time my son coughs or blinks too often—or anything—I blame myself. If I have another child I will never put him or me through that again. I want to do everything right."

Danger Signs in Early Pregnancy

Both now and later on in your pregnancy there are a number of symptoms which, because they do merit concern, should be reported to your physician when and if they occur: Vaginal bleeding, other than the slight staining that often occurs in the first few weeks, is always a source of concern. Ongoing headache, dimness or blurring of vision, severe abdominal pain, very frequent vomiting, a very high fever (over 101 for more than a day), or puffiness of the hands and face (this is of greater concern later on) should also signal a need for immediate medical attention.

CHAPTER 3

Growing

(Month 3)

THE PSYCHOLOGICAL

Telling Others

By the time you reach your third month, you will probably start informing your parents, other relatives, friends, and business associates, if you haven't done so already, that you are expecting a child. You should be aware that since parenthood is a time of transition, not only for the two of you but for people around you, from the moment others find out that you are prospective parents, your relationship with them will change at least somewhat—perhaps for the better, perhaps for the worse. Their reaction to your announcement may surprise you, may be very different from what you expected, and this difference could serve to improve or threaten your mutual feelings about each other.

Parents

Your expectations of how your mother and father and in-laws would react when they got the news was probably one which included gasps of joy, toasts to the new generation, and a great deal of general exuberance and merriment.

Perhaps this did (or will) happen, and you may have derived a great deal of pleasure out of watching them react. "We held off telling our parents because we wanted to make sure I was really pregnant and beyond the miscarriage phase," a blond 25-year-old former stewardess revealed. "It was so frustrating to have this incredible feeling of joy which you couldn't share with someone you loved. I kept hoping my mother would say, 'Gee, you're getting fat,' so I could respond, 'Oh Mom, it's only baby fat!'; or have her accuse me of 'letting yourself go,' and I'd come back with the line, 'Three months pregnant is *not* letting myself go!'

"But that was all part of my fantasy. When it came time to tell them, my husband and I went to their house for the weekend. I was looking a bit heavy at the time, and my mother announced that she was putting me on a diet right there and then. No breakfast, cottage cheese for lunch, and a carrot for dinner. She was serious! And then I told her. She immediately ran out to the store to fill the refrigerator with food, and when she came home, said, 'Eat! Eat! Don't starve my grandchild!' "

Another woman related another very happy "telling" experience: "I had it all figured out, I mean, how I was going to break the big news to our parents. We had all four of them over for dinner and I served them cheesecake for dessert, but placed a large bowl of pickles topped with ice cream at my place and said, 'Any questions?' Our two sets of parents started congratulating each other. They were all so excited."

Probably at least half the time, there is a great deal of happiness. But if you have long anticipated the pleasure of informing parents of your pregnancy, perhaps even imagining well before the conception what that moment would be like, it can come as a bit of a letdown to find out that they are not behaving exactly as you had planned.

"Instead of shrieking with delight, my mother started berating us for waiting so long," one new mother complained, laughing and shaking her head at the same time. "And my mother-in-law simply said, 'Are you kidding? Could you be serious? I was resigned to having cats and dogs and Teddy bears as my only grandchildren.' "

"It really hurt a bit when they greeted our news with, 'Well, it's about time,' " another expectant father confessed. "We had been trying for years to have a child and it finally happened—with a great deal of medical help, I might add. They made the wrong assumptions about how we felt about kids, thought we were just selfishly avoiding the responsibility."

Sometimes the circumstances are such that your news, while the most significant event which has ever happened in your life, is hardly a novelty to them, or can reopen old conflicts you have with parents or in-laws. "I had the feeling that my in-laws viewed my enlarging abdomen as just another baby-sitting assignment," a pregnant high school teacher commented somewhat bitterly. "My husband has two sisters who already had presented their mother with two grandchildren each, well before we were married. Of course, we knew that, but still, her lack of enthusiasm disappointed us because we wanted everyone to be as happy as we were."

Or, unfortunately, the announcement that a child is expected can come as a not totally welcome surprise to the prospective grandparents. "We were living together for three years before I conceived," a 23-year-old new mother reported. "My parents knew about it, but never would openly acknowledge it. When I was three months pregnant we went to their home for the weekend. We told them Friday night and they were very subdued, even though we explained that the pregnancy was planned and we intended to get married. They even stuck to their house rules, making us sleep in separate bedrooms because we weren't married!"

"My own mother was so thrilled to hear about the baby," a 25-year-old nursing student told me, "that it was quite a contrast to see how his mother reacted. I got the feeling she was brooding over the fact that we were having a child so soon after we got married, while my husband was still in graduate school. It was as if she viewed our announcement as just another burden on her son." She paused for a moment and reflected, "I wonder if the expectant paternal grandparents are ever really as excited as the parents of the mother. Somehow the biological tie may seem closer for my parents than it is for his."

"I was frankly astounded at the way my mother took the news," a 22-year-old woman in her ninth month whispered to me as her mother prepared coffee in the next room. "She's 50 years old and apparently going through some type of identity crisis right now. Being a grandmother seemed not to fit into her self-image. She's the type of woman who has always been so sensitive about her age that she probably claims her two grown children are older than she is!" She laughed, then continued, this time more seriously, "I knew she was like that, but it still hurt me that she didn't tell her friends right away that we were expecting." Her face brightened again. "But now she's getting very excited."

The designation "grandmother" does bring to mind a kindly little old lady in a rocking chair, with her hair in a bun, muffins in the oven, and knitting needles in her hands. So, understandably, some middle-aged women are a bit unsettled to be precipitously moved up the generational ladder at a time when they feel young and vibrant. And they might well be worried about the teasing they might get from others. ("I feel comfortable about becoming a grandfather," one 60-year-old man once told his wife, "but what I'm really concerned about is being married to a grandmother!") It can take

time for both sets of parents to get used to the idea, and the failure
to be overjoyed immediately by your announcement may reflect
that the transition to their new status is still in process.

Pregnancy and the months immediately after the birth can be a
particular stress point in a mother-daughter relationship. You may
find that you need your mother emotionally more than ever before
in your adult life. If your mother is not alive, living far away, or simply emotionally unavailable, you may miss her very much at this
time, and find yourself actively looking for someone to replace her.
Or you may discover that you and your mother have considerable
difficulty getting along on occasion, experiencing problems in determining exactly who is the mother and who is the child. "I was hesitant to tell my mother I was pregnant," a woman with a five-month-
old son in her lap told me. "I knew as soon as she found out, she'd
want to be in charge. She couldn't seem to accept the fact that this
baby was ours, not hers."

This type of reaction, and interpretation of things your mother—
or mother-in-law—says soon after she learns of your pregnancy,
may indeed reflect some new feelings on her part, or could be the
result of your increased sensitivity to the subject and all the implica-
tions of being pregnant. Angela Barron MacBride, in her book *The
Growth and Development of Mothers,* describes her sensitivity,
specifically how her own uncertainty about what it was going to be
like being a mother, shaded her interpretations of the gestures of
others. Her mother-in-law gave her a subscription to *Reader's
Digest* as a birthday gift after learning of her pregnancy, and Angela
thought, "Is she trying to tell me that I will not have the time, or
maybe the inclination, to read whole books once I am a mother?"

"My relationship with my parents regressed tremendously," a
child psychologist explained. "When I announced I was pregnant—
I was 30 at the time, well established in my own life and career—my
parents wanted to treat me like a child again. They began telling me
what I could and could not do. After years of leaving me on my own,
they suddenly felt responsible for me once more. My mother was
about to have me hospitalized one day, just because I sneezed. And
my father became furious at me when he saw me carrying two
loaded grocery bags into the house."

"The strangest thing happened when I told my mother that I was expecting," another woman volunteered. "She had for years been encouraging us to have kids, telling us how great it was. Then right after we told her I was pregnant, she started telling me about how sloppy babies were, how I used to spatter cereal all over the living room, how she didn't sleep through one night for a year after I was born, and on and on and on . . ."

On the other hand, you may find that your pregnancy and becoming a mother yourself brings you and your parents—particularly your mother—closer than ever before, perhaps because you have so much more in common. "It was amazing," a 30-year-old mother of two told me. "We simply never got along. But as soon as I conceived she was so kind, so solicitous of me. As I gradually realized how motherhood would change my life, I began to appreciate her efforts a bit more."

There is a Japanese proverb which says, "To understand parents' love, you must have a child of your own." For this woman, pregnancy helped her begin to understand her mother more and thus markedly improved their relationship.

As so often is the case with all transitions in life, where one is becoming accustomed to a new rank with new responsibilities and new privileges, understanding is the key. Realize that your parents are going through a type of crisis too (one which you also will probably experience someday). The first few months of pregnancy can be a testing point in the relationship you have with your parents and to emerge successfully you must learn to maintain a precarious balance, beginning to play the role of parent to your own child, while, to some extent, at least, remaining the child of your own parents.

Friends, Business Associates

If you are thrilled to be expecting a baby, you certainly expect your close friends to express the same sentiments. And in the majority of cases they will. "My girl friends knew that we had been trying, and I know they were genuinely pleased for me," a woman who had just started "telling" about her pregnancy explained. "I told them at a dinner party we had the other night, and they wanted to pamper me every moment after that, not letting me pick up even one dish to carry to the kitchen. And I know they were sincere."

Cornelia Otis Skinner once wrote, "A lady's announcement to her girl friends that she is going to do what, after all, quite a number of other women have done before—namely, give birth to a child—is a signal for them all to burst into tears." And, just as she wrote, that frequently does happen.

They may tease you in a friendly manner. ("Let's see, that means you were pregnant when we were at the beach house last month, and you didn't tell us!" Or, "So, you're starting a family after eight years of marriage. Sure you can make the transition?")

But sometimes the news is received with mixed emotions, or coolly. "Our best friends were dividing at the time we started to multiply," one woman explained, "and our great happiness did not go over well as they broke up their families." "My college roommate wasn't married then—and I knew she wished she were," another new mother commented. "I guess it was too much for her to see that I appeared to have everything she wanted. We haven't heard from her since. She kind of dropped out."

"I think I can understand that," another pregnant woman who overheard these comments admitted. "When we were postponing pregnancy, working hard and saving money, a number of my college friends would call and gleefully announce their condition. It would depress me. I really began to wonder if we would ever have even one baby, whether the circumstances would ever be right for us. I tried to act happy, but there were times that not having something I wanted hurt me a lot."

Other childfree friends may feel that your announcement means they are losing your companionship, that the old gang is breaking up. Or they might actually act hostile, responding with, "I can't believe you are having a child," or "Well, I hope this means you'll be giving up your job," a comment that suggests that since they don't have both, you shouldn't either.

You may well find that your friends who have children are much more outspoken and sincere in their expressions of joy and well-wishing than are those without children, perhaps because they simply have more in common with you now or have no reason to be threatened by your news. Couples with children may react with comments like, "Welcome to a new world of incredible joy and tenderness," or they may appear to take great pleasure in telling you,

"Boy, if you only knew what you were in for," relating more details of their own pregnancy and early days of parenthood than you really care to hear about. "I found that most women were reasonably restrained about their labor and delivery experiences," was the way one newly expectant mother put it. "But when I told my friends our news I heard the agonies of this and the misery of that. And the funny thing was I got the feeling that they were a bit envious that it was me, not them, suddenly in this chamber of horrors!"

Indeed, friends and relatives may say some very odd things to you, as exemplified by the story of a 25-year-old mother-to-be: "Right after my husband told his best friend, he came over to the house and pulled me aside, saying, 'Look, Gail, don't hold it against John if he isn't too interested in sex with you while you are carrying the baby. You know men do wander during this time, but it's nothing to be upset about.' Well, I was furious, let me tell you!"

While you may be eager to tell parents and friends of your condition as soon as you feel that it's "safe," you may be less eager to tell those you work with. "I told only one woman at work," a research assistant at an advertising agency confided to me, "and she advised me not to tell our boss until it became obvious. Well, I put on weight fast and in the middle of my third month she came in to my office and whispered, 'It's obvious!' I told the boss and his reaction was, 'How could you *do* this to me?' He offered his best wishes and everything but despite the fact that I explained how I planned to work up until my ninth month and would return within two months after the baby came, I could tell that he felt he could no longer count on me. I ended up working twice as hard during my pregnancy, just to prove to him I was able to hang in there."

"I was hesitant about approaching the principal at my school," a junior high school teacher recalled. "When I did tell him, he acted as though it shouldn't change my role there at all. But the next day at a teachers' meeting he made a reference to my 'not being there next month because I would be having a baby.' I was three months pregnant at the time."

Expectant fathers may be hesitant or actually eager to inform their associates at work. "If my boss at the bank knew," one man in an executive training program explained, "he would conclude that I was in an economically pressured situation, afraid to leave the job no matter what promotion they passed me up on. I wanted to keep my image as a footloose and childfree employee as long as possible." "Not me," said another expectant father after I told him about this man's reaction. "I felt that the fact I was going to be a father was good news for my career. It gave me more of a stable image. I looked forward to having the mother and baby picture on my desk. And I feel my boss greeted the news very approvingly."

Of course your employer and the people you work with may be enthusiastic, offering you all types of advice on how to have a successful pregnancy, and the worst you'll have to endure is being called "little momma" or some variation on that theme. Your relationship with men in the office may actually improve. Virginia Barber and Merrill Skaggs, in their book *A Mother Person*, write that some women feel men find them less threatening, more approachable, when they are pregnant.

You may inform your business associates in a straightforward way that you are pregnant, telling that you are due around "X" date and that you do or do not plan to work up to that date and after the birth. Or you may be more circumspect, avoiding the issue until you are well into the pregnancy, or until you may feel you have to. If you think you are being unjustly discriminated against at work because you are pregnant, speak up. Such stereotyping of pregnant women is no longer appropriate, if it ever was. But on the other hand, be fair to your employer, too. Be honest about the date you intend to leave and whether you will be cutting back on work hours before and immediately after the birth.

When you contemplate telling your friends and associates of your pregnancy, no matter what type of reaction you expect, consider a rule discovered too late for a number of prospective parents: don't be impatient with your meager beginnings. Don't overstate how pregnant you are just so they will think it is "real." If you do, you'll regret it later! One woman who learned from experience explained, "When I was seven weeks pregnant I told my friends I was three months along, expecting in June. I thought it sounded more significant that way! Well, when June came, the phone never stopped ringing. Finally I had to confess to them that my due date was July 15th."

Couples who are expecting a second child frequently report that their concern with the reaction and acceptance of their pregnancy is almost exclusively centered on the child they have, rather than any relative or friend. Certainly the circumstances under which you will tell your child are determined to a great extent on how old he or she is. But in any case you'll probably want to pick a time when there is not a great deal of emotional commotion already in the child's life—not, for example, during the first week of school or an intensive period of toilet training. But whatever the occasion you eventually choose—don't postpone it until too late in pregnancy. A few books for expectant parents suggest that you wait until the child sees a bulging abdomen and then begins to ask. "No good!" was the way one mother of three evaluated that advice. "Almost from the beginning they hear you discussing it and then there's always some clod on the elevator who says to the child, 'Say, I hear you're going to have a baby brother pretty soon.' They have to be told early. There are some excellent children's books that help explain it all."

Feeling Different

The Highs, the Lows

Pregnant women see and react to things differently than do nonpregnant women. While cartoons and articles in women's magazines frequently overstate the eccentricity of expectant mothers, "emotional lability," or in everyday language, frequent mood variation, is a psychological characteristic of the pregnant state. Under old English law, a pregnant woman's testimony was not accepted in court because she was considered unreliable. Like the cartoons and stories, this exaggerates the situation, but, nevertheless, it does underscore the point that ups and downs are common and have affected women for generations.

Why does this emotional lability occur? Presumably, hormonal influences have a significant influence. Progesterone is produced in increasing amounts once conception occurs, and one of the characteristics of this hormone is a depressing effect. There is also evidence that corticosteroid hormone levels (hormones secreted mainly by the adrenal glands) are altered during pregnancy.

But an altered chemical environment is not all that is involved. Pregnancy is a major transition, and you'll likely alternate for a while between a wish for the future with a baby and the wish for the past when you were independent, without the responsibility for a dependent child. "There were a few moments," Joan, a professional dancer in her early twenties, commented, "when I began to remember how low, how exhausted some of my friends were after their babies were born. And how their lives changed, how tied down they were. I kept thinking, 'Oh my God, what if that happens to me? Is it too late to change my mind?' I really needed the full nine months to work out all those conflicts."

"Do you know what made me low?" another woman in mid-pregnancy asked. "When I was about three months pregnant I began imagining that the worst would happen, that I'd have a deformed child, that everything would go wrong, that the whole thing would be a terrible mistake. Last night I had a nightmare along the lines of a movie I once saw, one where a woman gave birth and the baby, as soon as it was born, began killing people in the delivery room. Then the next day I read somewhere that if you worry too much while you carry a boy he might turn out to be a homosexual, and that made me worry even more."

The anxieties of early pregnancy are often manifest in dreams (other women have reported dreaming that they gave birth to dogs, horses, or monkeys at this stage), and in daytime transient depression.

"I was perfectly cheerful, enjoying being pregnant," a 23-year-old new mother told me, "until in the middle of my third month when I passed a hospital emergency room and saw a mother carrying her three- or four-year-old child out of an ambulance. I was depressed for days over that. Later on in my pregnancy I read a newspaper account of a child abuse incident and I had a similar sick-to-my-stomach feeling."

"I'd say my current low is the fact that I'm exhausted all the time," many women in their third month complain. "Sometimes I think my mind is going," added one. "I get into bed in the afternoon and listen to the radio. It's getting so I know the weatherman's name on every station."

Small family arguments, a minor exchange of harsh words which, in other circumstances would be quickly forgotten or ignored, can be enough to set off a flood of tears. "My husband made a sarcastic comment about the casserole I made last week," Sandra, in her third month of pregnancy, confided to me. "I immediately ran into the bedroom and cried for an hour. He didn't know what to do with me. And a few times during the last weeks I've gotten very resentful that his life was proceeding as usual, while my pace was slowing down. I've become a bit snappy and when he responds in kind, I just collapse in tears."

"Last week my husband was talking about his brother's new baby," another woman sheepishly admitted, "and I was very hurt—to the point of tears—that he was talking about someone else's baby, not ours. I know it was ridiculous, but there I was crying."

The highs and lows during pregnancy affect the expectant father too. He may be very pleased by the new demands you place on him if they are not too great, his self-esteem increasing as he begins to feel more protective of you. Or he may feel low, unnecessarily burdened, especially if you are assuming an "I am pregnant, now take care of me" attitude. Concerns about whether or not he really wants to be present at the delivery of the child—an issue you may already have made up your mind about—or down-to-earth, practical worries about supporting a larger family may be responsible for his lows. "I had just turned 25 when Mary became pregnant," one new father recalled. "I felt like a child myself. It took me about six months of the pregnancy even to begin to feel comfortable with that kind of responsibility."

"My most vulnerable point," another new father explained, "was the fact that I simply felt totally out of it. My wife seemed increasingly to be interested in herself and her body. I got the feeling there was no role for me between fertilizing the egg and handing out the cigars. I'm the type that likes to be a player, not a spectator, so it was frustrating. I had to try very hard to get her attention, and our sex life was almost nonexistent. She was always too tired."

"Frankly, I had a lot of second thoughts," another expectant father told me. "During those early months of pregnancy when I saw kids in the playground behind our apartment, I thought to myself, 'You mean, I've actually got to learn to *like* them?' "

The normal emotional lability of pregnancy will, of course, be intensified if there is still any sense of serious conflict in you, your husband or both, about the desirability of the pregnancy. "My husband was stunned when I told him I was pregnant, and not very pleased at all. For the first three months he seemed to bury himself in his work and I felt very, very alone. The only thing that kept me going was my absolute confidence that the baby would win him over as soon as he or she was born."

Your Changing Body Image

"I wanted to be noticed right away," Judy, a 25-year-old secretary in her fifth month, exclaimed to me as we chatted in the lunchroom in her office. "I began looking for maternity clothes as soon as I got the test results. And I could hardly wait until I had even the slightest reason to abandon my regular clothes. By the time I was two and a half months along I told friends I couldn't get my zippers to go up—which wasn't exactly true. I've always been envious of pregnant women I see on the street. I just love the way I look now."

Ellen, a 23-year-old graduate student, had a very different reaction as she began her third month of pregnancy. "I've always made an effort to keep slim. I don't like bulges or generally fat people. Now I'm beginning to have the feeling I am living beyond my seams—and maternity clothes with those kangaroo-like pouches in front really turn me off."

We all have an image of our bodies, how we like to look. Given that the third month of pregnancy brings with it a variety of physical changes, some of which can be noticed by people who know you well, your image of yourself may change, for better or worse. You, like Judy, may be eager to have the world know of your condition, walking with your shoulders high, rigidly back so your abdomen protrudes. Even before the buttons on your blouse show signs of strain, you may be wearing, as one maternity shop advertised, "peachy clothes for pear-shaped ladies." You may think you look terrific. Or you may not feel comfortable at all about your image in this in-between stage where people look at you slightly puzzled and obviously a bit suspicious. "I've been looking for one of those sweatshirts that says, 'I'm not fat, I'm just pregnant,' " a number of expectant mothers in this in-between phase told me.

You may try to pass as long as you can, choosing selectively from your regular wardrobe for loose-fitting clothes. Or perhaps, as another new mother recollected, "Some days I just wanted to be like my nonpregnant self. But there were other days when I was three months pregnant that I definitely wanted to brag about it."

Some of the physical changes may please you immensely. "I felt voluptuous for the first time in my life," a petite saleswoman told me. "My breasts became full right away and stayed that way during the entire pregnancy. By the time I was in my ninth month people were accusing me of carrying the baby in my bust."

The extraordinary physical changes that will occur in your body take some getting used to. It can be emotionally unsettling to feel that you really are out of control of those changes, unable to go on a crash diet to become slim again. If you are used to being slender, the fullness of your body may simply be uncomfortable and you may cringe at the slight, but to you noticeable, expansion of your waistline. You may be curious, fascinated by the physical happenings. "I began to see veins I never even knew I had," one woman exclaimed. "I read a great deal about the incredible growth of the fetus by the third month and I was fascinated to look at my body and think that all that was going on with just a minimum of change in my outward appearance."

THE PHYSICAL

By the beginning of the third month your growing child's face is completely formed; arms, legs, hands, and feet partially so. Many of the organs, already there in primitive form, begin to specialize in function. For example, during these weeks the third and final kidney stage forms and begins to function, the finishing touch to be added after birth. If a microscopic examination could be performed at this point (which it can't, at least not on a currently pregnant woman) the sex of the baby would be known, as the sex glands have already appeared. Indeed, in the course of these first three months the basic development of the child has occurred; changes after that are more subtle, simply a matter of enlargement and maturation of the various organs. At three months of age your baby is about six and a half inches long and weighs about one-quarter of a pound.

Eating Right

It is in the third month that your nutritional needs begin to change. But contrary to what you might have heard (and perhaps hoped for), you do not need significantly greater quantities of food while you are pregnant.

The National Academy of Sciences recommends that a typical woman 5'5", normally weighing about 128 pounds, requires approximately 2100 calories a day when she is not pregnant, or one to two months pregnant; 2400 when she is three or more months pregnant; and 2600–2800 when she is breast feeding. As already mentioned in Chapter 2, you can get your 2400 calories in well-balanced form by having 2–4 glasses of skim milk; 2 servings of meat, chicken, or fish; 1 egg; 4 servings of fruits and vegetables (including citrus, dark green, leafy, or yellow vegetables); 4 servings from the bread and cereal category, each day. Again, you do not have to eat *more* food to meet the needs of pregnancy—you just must make sure you follow the "variety and balance" rule. Unfortunately, it is difficult to follow this rule and stay within the calorie limit if you attempt to include nonnecessary food items like rich desserts, mayonnaise, salad dressings—or (although they are not technically foods) cocktails.

Your doctor has probably told you that during your entire pregnancy you should put on no more than a total of 23–26 pounds, and that the weight should be gained primarily during the fifth to ninth months. You may come to despise the scale in his office and on more than one occasion will be tempted to "cheat" on the reading when the nurse isn't looking. For the past fifty years obstetricians have been encouraging patients to limit their weight gain—sometimes severely. Early in the century the advice had some very immediate, practical applications: given that there is a relationship between the baby's birth weight and the amount of weight the mother gains, and since large babies often presented obstetrical complications, caloric restriction was essential. More recently, however, the advice about weight control was based on the theory that excessive weight gain led to acute toxemia of pregnancy. Today this theory is no longer accepted and the strict warnings which you routinely receive as you step off the scale are related more to *your* general health and the knowledge that for many American women, lifetime weight problems begin with pregnancy.

Your attempt to keep your diet balanced and stay within reasonable calorie boundaries may be threatened to some extent by that almost exclusive-to-pregnancy phenomenon known as the "food craving."

If you raise the subject with most new mothers, you'll find that they are as eager to tell you about what their individual food craving was ("With Jeffrey it was jelly doughnuts, with Amy I was suddenly crazy for steak," or "I simply couldn't get enough Chinese food . . .") as they are to tell you all the details of their labor and delivery.

The reason for the cravings is not well understood, but they have for years been observed in pregnant women. (In England expectant mothers are often referred to as being in a "longing way.") Simone de Beauvoir in *The Second Sex* writes about a woman who had such a mad desire for spinach that she ran to the market to buy it, tapping her foot impatiently at home while it cooked. A woman related a similar type of "emergency" incident to me: "I was doing research in the library, going over old women's magazines, and suddenly I saw an ad for Oreo cookies. I never eat cookies of any type, but the urge to have one was so strong, I had to leave the library right away and buy a box. I ate them right in the store."

Perhaps there is some biological cause for food cravings,[1] but more likely it is a psychological phenomenon of wanting to indulge yourself, or perhaps using food to allay any fears and anxieties that confront you at the moment. While you might say "absolutely ridiculous" to the notion of strawberry shortcake at 4 A.M. when you are not pregnant, you may now think, "Well, I guess it's okay, considering my condition."

Unless food cravings truly get out of control, either by straining your budget (a continued desire for lobster can definitely have this effect), or by precluding a well-balanced, moderate diet, these cravings should not be a source of concern. After all, they are almost a matter of tradition.

Pregnancy Symptoms in Men?

Psycholanalysts tell us that men really want to be pregnant. They note that in Greek mythology, Zeus carries Dionysus sewed up in his thigh until ripe for birth, and that Athena's birth from the head of Zeus is a symbol of the procreative push for men.

They might also note the example of nineteenth-century author Dostoevsky's reactions during his second wife's first pregnancy. He was then married to his stenographer, 25 years younger than he, after having been a widower for three years and having no children by the first marriage. During the first six months of the pregnancy, he avoided work on his projected novel, *The Idiot.* He later maintained that of all the novels he created, this was the most difficult for him. He recalled his frustration in attempting to write: "The idea I have is so good, and so pregnant with meaning, that I worship it.

---

1. Some scientists have recently suggested that the common cravings for sweets during pregnancy leads to a sweetening of the amniotic fluid, causing the fetus to drink more of it.

And yet what will come of it? I know beforehand I'll work on it for eight or nine months and I'll make a mess of it. Two or three years are necessary for something of this kind."

Do men wish to be pregnant? And, whether or not they have this wish, do they experience side effects of pregnancy, much the way their wives do? There is some evidence that about 10 to 20 percent of husbands do suffer from loss of appetite, heartburn, toothache, or nausea at this time. These symptoms are reminiscent of an ancient primitive ritual called "couvade," a form of "sympathetic magic" where the husband goes to bed complaining of abdominal pains during the time his wife is in labor. Perhaps these symptoms reflect the man's desire somehow to be part of an experience he was very much involved in initiating. Or perhaps he is more aware of these symptoms—and more likely to be teased by others—at this time in his life.

CHAPTER 4

The Middle Trimester

(Months 4, 5, and 6)

THE PSYCHOLOGICAL

Feeling Good

Many Highs

> *Everyone told me that I'd feel terrific once I got over the first three months, and they were right! My complexion glows, my hair shines, and it's thicker than ever. I like my body now. I definitely look pregnant, but I'm not so big that it's uncomfortable to move around.*
>
> —Gloria, 24-year-old housewife, fourth month

> *I feel well, but also quite different at the same time. I'm emotionally in high gear. I'm sensitive, very aware of everything that's going on. It's as though the volume on life is tuned higher than normal.*
>
> —Annette, 33-year-old laboratory technician, fifth month

> *At other times in my life I've often been chilled, shivering, running for a sweater. But right now I feel very warm inside, as if I'm glowing. And that keeps me very comfortable.*
>
> —Ellen, 27-year-old college instructor, fifth month

> *We worried for years about whether or not to have children. It was a tremendous source of inner pressure, fearing that a baby would disrupt our busy lives, yet at the same time very anxious that we'd be making a terrible mistake by not having at least one. Now we have the best of both worlds. She feels great and looks terrific. Our sex life has never been better. We're closer than ever before. The pressure is off. We're going to have a baby, but we don't have any of the responsibilities yet."*
>
> —Albert, 36, a freelance writer, wife in fourth month

As these expectant parents illustrate, the middle months of pregnancy are often the high point psychologically and physically. The
nausea of the early months has probably passed. The look of being
slightly plump has changed into a definitely pregnant appearance.
You're excited, anticipating, yet far enough away from delivery that
you needn't be concerned about a things-to-do-at-the-last-minute
list. The emotional lability of pregnancy is still with you, but you are
not overwhelmed by it and perhaps occasionally laugh at yourself
when you feel tears coming for no legitimate reason.

Ellen's comment about feeling warm recalls an observation that
one of psychoanalyst Dr. Helene Deutsch's pregnant patients once
made: "It is like a stove in the winter that is always lit, that is there
for you alone, entirely subject to your will. It is also like a constantly
gushing cold shower in the summer, refreshing you. It is there."

"I simply loved the way she looked, as soon as she began to
show," an expectant father told me as he put his arm around his
wife, then nine months pregnant. "I thought she looked incredibly
sexy. I used to take pictures of her every week, starting about the
fourth month, to go with the diary of events she was keeping. When
I came home after a rough day at the office I got an instant lift when
I saw her bulge. 'Now that's something to live for,' I would tell
myself."

"We were very future-oriented during those months," another
new father recalled. "So much of what we would say to each other
was prefaced by 'when the baby comes.' Those months were when
we made arrangements for our new apartment, thought about fixing
up the baby's room." He paused. "We were a bit uneasy about that!
It was so strange to be making arrangements for someone who
wasn't born yet. We were both a bit superstitious about buying
things at that point, so we just wrote down the model numbers and
ordered them later."

Of course, feeling good doesn't always translate out to feeling full
or productive energy. Indeed, many women report that during
most of pregnancy, but particularly during the middle months, they
feel sluggish, in a dreamlike state, unable to accomplish very much.
In their book *The Mother Person*, Virginia Barber and Merrill
Skaggs, while acknowledging that the middle months can be a
"high," note the reaction of a painter who declared, "I don't think I

had a single fresh idea during my entire pregnancy." The authors add: "And her words were echoed by many women who felt dull, almost drugged. Few said that this new life evolving inside them brought on a burst of mental creativity; just the reverse. The body with its changing and insistent demands tends to overwhelm any other urges."

Quickening

Somewhere between the sixteenth and twenty-second weeks of pregnancy you will become aware that the child in your uterus is not only alive and growing, but moving as well. This usually occurs earlier in a woman who is having a second or later child, later for the first-time mother—but don't worry if it doesn't follow this exact schedule.

Movement may start as a flicker, a wiggly feeling—"like the flap of a fish," "the flutter of a bird" is how some characterize it. Adrienne Rich, in *Of Woman Born*, describes quickening this way: "In early pregnancy, the stirrings of the fetus felt like ghostly tremors of my own body, later like the movements of a being imprisoned in me." At first you may think it's your imagination or simply some intestinal gas, but within days you'll realize that neither of these has limbs.

To your chagrin, the moment of quickening is only detectable by you, not your husband, but it is a major landmark of pregnancy. (Leave it to the school of psychoanalysis to describe this emotional event in superscientific terms, referring to it as "the relevance of the productive interior . . . a sense of vital inner potential.") Generally this first detectable flutter represents the beginning of the transition from being primarily concerned with yourself and your own bodily changes, to focusing on the new, very individual life inside you.

"I hungered for some knowledge of what he or she was like, once I felt the flutter," a smiling woman in her fifth month told me. "It is very real now, but I still don't know who this person inside me is, what he or she is like."

As soon as she told me our baby was kicking, our relationship began to change," an expectant father explained. "Now there were three of us. We began talking to the baby, calling him 'Baby Bear.'

We would ask Baby Bear what he would like for dinner. And later, when the movement got particularly intense, my wife would say to me, 'Tell Baby Bear to stop kicking me!' "

A Few Lows: Emotional Problems of the Middle Months

"Feeling Life"

Sometimes advancing pregnancy, and particularly quickening, can have an unsettling, or at least sobering, effect. "When she told me the baby had kicked, I had a little of the same feeling as when I first learned she was pregnant," Sam, an expectant father whose wife was due any day, explained. "It made it so very real to hear this little thing was actually moving on its own. Before, I was obviously aware that we were expecting a child. But the movement, even though I couldn't feel it right then, removed any of the fantasy that might have been there."

"I was really very excited that day I felt the first kick," a 20-year-old new mother told me. "I remember I was working at my desk at the bank and I felt something like a noiseless beep. I pressed my hand into my stomach and this time it felt stronger. I knew that was it. It was exciting but frightening at the same time. I never had a living thing inside of me before! I think I realized then that this baby was his own person. That it was just using my body temporarily, like a parasite, and then would go on its own. I dreamed that night that right after the baby was born he joined the navy. That upset me a bit!"

Simone de Beauvoir wrote of quickening: "Women perceive the child's first movements with varied feelings, this kicking delivered at the portals of the world, against the uterine wall that shuts off the world. One woman is lost in wonder at this signal, announcing the presence of an independent being; another may feel repugnance at containing a stranger. Once more the union of fetus and maternal body is disturbed. . . . Up to this time he has been only a mental image, a hope; now he becomes a solid present reality, and this reality creates new problems."

Quickening *is* a major emotional event. It *can* be unsettling as well as exciting. You may well find that your immediate reaction is a nervous gulp rather than a cry of joy. It's just one of many landmarks of the pregnancy experience which can evoke a mixture of feelings, all of which are likely to fall into the "normal" category.

Obviously Pregnant

"As I was just starting my fourth month, I thought I could still pass," commented Janet, a real estate broker, as we chatted in her office. "I was initially upset when I realized how naive I was about this. One night at a restaurant the waiter brought a tray of desserts around. When I refused, he cajoled me, 'Oh come now, you're eating for two.' Then, the next day—again, I thought I was still looking relatively slim in my slacks and my husband's shirt worn over them—a grocery delivery boy came to the door, looked at me and asked 'Boy or girl?' " She laughed at the recollection, adding, "I was at first unnerved that my secret was no more."

"Right around that time I remember that people started giving me uneasy, uncertain looks," volunteered one of Janet's associates who had recently given birth and was listening to our conversation. "There was a time there when some of the people whom I hadn't told I was expecting were obviously uncomfortable. They didn't know whether to say, 'Oh, you're going to have a baby,' or to keep quiet in case I was just plain fat! If I get pregnant again, I think I'll tell people when I'm in that in-between stage so they aren't left just wondering and staring.

"Anyway," she continued, "by the fifth month I began to get some special treatment—like a bus seat. Or people would just smile knowingly at me. But, you know, I found it very difficult coming to terms with the fact that people on the street knew my condition. Even when I'm not pregnant I'm the type who feels exposed in the springtime when I don't have a coat. I prefer to wear one. And all through my middle and later months I wore a big coat, through the warmth of spring and the brutal heat of summer." She stopped, then spoke more quickly but with emphasis, "It's not that I didn't like my shape. I just didn't like sharing it with others."

Around the fourth month of pregnancy, it does become obvious to the world that you have joined the ranks of The Pregnant Women. Even if you are not generally a private type of person, the kind who doesn't want to share her thoughts and feelings with other than your closest friends and relatives, you may at this time begin to feel somewhat self-conscious when you're walking down the street, perhaps a bit annoyed, as Janet's associate was, that everyone "knew." As she mentioned, until you feel comfortable about going public— and you almost certainly will by the middle of your pregnancy—big coats and loose dresses can help.

Self-Centered and Introspective?

In your middle months you find yourself increasingly occupied with thoughts about the baby and your changing body. Since this may pose some problems in your relationship with others—your friends, associates, and your husband—you may want to examine critically your behavior and make changes as necessary, anticipating difficulties before they occur.

"One day when I was six months along," a petite and very pregnant beautician told me, "I was having lunch with a friend, chatting merrily away about this and that. My friend was very quiet. Finally she burst out, 'Don't you talk about anything except your pregnancy?' I was initially startled, then I realized that I was becoming a bit of a bore—tremendously self-centered."

This phase of pregnancy *can* be trying on those around you, and perhaps you can learn something from this woman's experience. When people ask "How are you?", chances are they probably don't want to hear every little detail of how your body is changing. While your friends obviously have some interest in hearing of your pregnancy, they probably would like to talk about other things too.

A sense of feeling left out because of your marked introspection can be at the basis of emotional difficulty for the expectant father. "She was so involved with herself!" was the complaint about the middle months offered by a number of fathers-to-be. Some men put it this way: "Her own little world was overcharged"; "She was on her own private trip while I just stood by and watched, a bit frustrated." Your husband's feelings may be very understandable. You probably have a developing relationship with your friends, relatives, and obstetrician—one which may not include him. And he may, simply stated, be jealous, fulfilling Sigmund Freud's prediction that a baby is a "husband's dangerous rival." The biological rules are inflexible. *You* are the one who is carrying the baby. But there are ways of getting your man more involved. Ask him how he feels, what his thoughts are about your pregnancy, what his image of the growing baby is, what his anxieties and hopes focus on. Include him in your decision making about labor, childbirth, breast feeding, planning the child's room.

"Harry simply loved to buy stuffed animals 'for the baby' all through my pregnancy," a mother of three recalled. "I was frequently upset, only because they were so expensive and a real burden on our budget. Then he came home with a five-foot-high musical teddy bear, I protested vehemently. He was very hurt and exclaimed, 'You know, it's my baby too!' I got the message and figured that was my cue to come out of my own world and let him get as much involved and in any way he wanted."

Too often pregnancy is just the first step in excluding or greatly limiting the role of the father throughout parenthood. "Experts" in the field are often no help. For example, John Bowlby, writing in 1951, stated that "[the father] is of no direct importance to the young child, but is of indirect value as an economic support and in his emotional support of the mother." This attitude beginning in pregnancy is no longer—and probably never was—appropriate. Don't become so introspective, so wrapped up in yourself that you exclude your husband from what is by definition half his.

Ambivalence

For the majority of couples, the middle months of pregnancy are relatively calm, passive, and peaceful, characterized by only relatively minor disturbances.

For example, you may have a fleeting feeling that you are now powerless over the events of your daily life, dominated by the life that is inside you.

"Both of us often felt that we were caught up in a series of events we no longer had control over," was the reaction I commonly heard. "We often thought longingly of our former life, realizing we were on a course which we couldn't reverse, even if we wanted to," was another similar reaction. Or you may occasionally have surges of serious regrets, especially the "What did I do with my life?" syndrome.

Marcy, a 32-year-old dress designer who had with her husband spent many years thinking through the question of whether or not to have children, was a bit unsettled when, in the middle of what she describes as "one of the world's best-planned pregnancies," she had some distrubing, although transient, second thoughts. "All my professional life I've been trying to get some television producer to ask me to take charge of a series on fashion design," she lamented. "Now, just as I'm starting my fifth month, a producer from an out-of-town station called and told me that if I could work intensely on a series for the next four months, they'd give me a contract. What terrible timing! It bothered me very much to have to turn down that assignment. And when I hung up the phone I asked myself, 'Why am I pregnant? Why am I messing up my life this way?' I was really startled to have those thoughts. I had no idea before I became pregnant how strong those feelings could be. They did pass, but at the time I considered myself quite abnormal."

She certainly should not have. After all, if in your prepregnancy days, and perhaps continuing now, you were involved in a career or other activities outside the home, it is very likely that your priorities are going to take some time to shift. All your other interests are not going to disappear the moment you find out you're pregnant. During your pregnancy experience and after the baby is born, you may have to turn down a number of opportunities—vacations, social events, or, as Marcy described, an interesting job assignment. And the fact that you feel somewhat resentful is not inconsistent with your basic desire to have a baby. This ambivalence is the type which is common following any major life decision where a number of attractive options are vying for your attention. You will always wonder about "the road not taken," and once in a while berate yourself for making "the wrong" decision.

Only very rarely does either of the expectant parents carry over to the seventh, eighth, or ninth month any significant resistance of the pregnancy. But sometimes in the middle months, the conflicts of early pregnancy remain. The overwhelming proportion of these problems involves a still reluctant, or apparently reluctant, expectant father.

Sometimes the conflicts are relatively minor, although the hurt you feel at the time is not. "I asked my husband to go shopping with me last weekend to pick out some nursery things," one woman complained. "He got as far as the infant department, saw one crib, and announced he'd wait for me in the lobby. Why? Because he said the baby things 'depressed' him. I was very hurt at that moment. I asked myself, 'Does that mean he really isn't happy about our child?' " She smiled, then went on, "But I'm too excited myself to be depressed by that—I know he will come around soon."

But in a few cases the continued lack of support from an expectant father can be emotionally devastating. "When I was five months pregnant I still didn't feel that Jim was happy about the baby," Alice, a social worker in her late twenties and now the mother of a three-month-old girl, told me, "and let me make it very clear that I was very low.

"I think part of it was that he ignored me sexually at a time when I was very interested, very turned on, very physically oriented. But there was more. He was so distant, offering me none of the little things I expected during pregnancy—like holding my arm on the icy street so I wouldn't slip. He seemed to be in his own world. On a few nights I would cry so hard that I began to worry if it could harm the baby." She stopped, pushed her hair back and went on, speaking more slowly, "I even thought about a woman in John Updike's novel, *Couples*. She was very pregnant and very depressed and went out and had an affair to cheer herself up. I decided, 'I'll go out and have an affair; that will make him sorry!' But then I looked at my body and thought, 'Who would want me like this?' " She shook her head sadly. "The thing that kept me going was the fact that we basically did have a good relationship. And I knew the pregnancy would end eventually and there would be brighter horizons ahead of us."

A few days after this conversation I spoke with Alice's husband, Jim, to hear his side of the story. "I agree. I wasn't as supportive as I should have been. I simply couldn't get enthusiastic about a child I wasn't sure I wanted, didn't know anything about, a baby that might bring chaos to our lives. I was simply so uncertain. But I think she overstates the situation. Sometimes I got the feeling that she would look for support from me when she was feeling uncertainty about having a child. And if I wasn't superenthusiastic enough to compensate for her doubts at the moment, she interpreted it as meaning I didn't want the baby."

He stopped, took a deep breath, and sat back in his chair, speaking more softly. "When I look at the beautiful little girl we have right now I think, 'Why did I ever hesitate? Why didn't I make the pregnancy really great for both of us?' " He paused again, this time to change topics. "Oh, about the absence of our sex life, which I know she mentioned. Part of it was that I spent more time than ever at my job, a sort of distraction from my worries, I guess. And I was tired. Another part was I really didn't know if it was all right to have sex. I'm not the type who reads medical guides on sexuality, so I concluded that it was better not to take the chance. Beyond that, we weren't communicating the way we usually do. Things were very tense between us. It was like we both were waiting for the pregnancy to be over, the baby to be with us, so that we could then go on with our lives. I know expectant fathers, many of them still hesitant, will be reading your book. All I can say to them is that I was there and it's very different once the baby is born. The attachment you feel right away is amazing; the surge of emotion they evoke, breathtaking. 'Have confidence'—that's about the only advice I can offer. And, above all, communicate with each other. Don't build the emotional barrier we did."

If your husband is still, in your opinion, unenthusiastic about your pregnancy, perhaps you both might benefit from the comments Jim offered, or by the findings of Dr. Kay Standley, a psychologist who has studied pregnancy at the National Institute of Health. As a result of her work, Dr. Standley concluded that most men are truly interested in their wives' pregnancies and that the apparent lack of support and involvement masks their own anxiety. While there is certainly no guaranteed formula for handling this problem you might encourage your husband to talk with you about his concerns, and share your own with him. In short, as Jim suggested, communicate!

Coping with Realities

"Before we decided to have the baby we talked about how we were going to keep our old lives intact," a 34-year-old buyer for one of the large New York stores, now in her seventh month, related to me. "We agreed that I shouldn't quit my job. I'm making a good salary and enjoy my work. We decided to get help and stay in our current apartment. You know, when you wait to have kids, too much change in lifestyle all at once isn't good." She shook her head. "Now all out plans seem to be falling apart. Everything all of a sudden seems complicated. We were so naive! Our apartment is too small. Where am I going to find help? My God, should I really go right back to work after the baby is born? All at once we have all these questions to face, ones we thought we had long since settled."

A very common realization of mid-pregnancy is that you are at the point where issues which were in the "for the future" pile are now up for immediate attention. The reaction that the woman above had is not unusual at all. There *are* a lot of things to be settled. You may have to move and realize now that if a change of residence is required, you'd better do it soon, before you are simply too big to be carried over a new threshold. If you plan to continue working once the baby has arrived, it might be a good time to think of possibilities of day care help (you probably can wait until your eighth or ninth month to begin interviewing if you are going to hire a baby nurse or other type of helper).

Deal with the questions one at a time as they come up, and do everything you can to avoid having them overwhelm you. Some might be easily handled or delegated. Maybe your friends or parents might help you in your search for second-hand baby furniture. Others will require more thought and reflection which can only be done by the two of you. For example, the question of whether or not to return to work after the child is born is something only you can answer.

For the past few decades there has been heated debate over the question of whether it is psychologically necessary for the child to have the mother in full-time attendance. There probably isn't any professional child specialist today who would insist that a baby or young child needs his mother or one parent every waking moment.

In fact, most all psychiatrists and psychologists emphatically stress the rule: "Get out. Get some help so you can have a life of your own!" But even those who are very open-minded on the question of working mothers are not enthusiastic about an immediate return to work. The have-a-baby-and-go-back-to-the-fields approach might indeed interfere with the attachment phases. Dr. Mary C. Howell of Massachusetts General Hospital, who has closely examined the impact a working mother has on her child's development, concludes that there are "no uniformly harmful effects on family life," but adds that "a mother should return to work gradually, and only when she feels that she and the baby are ready to leave their exceptionally intimate postpartum relationship." This is a question that the two of you will want to consider, and possibly leave open-ended to see how you feel in the first weeks after your baby is born.

THE PHYSICAL

By the beginning of the fifth month, you almost certainly can feel the fetal movements and can hear the baby's heartbeat when your doctor shares the stethoscope with you. The baby is in a supine position with the head lower than the feet. The skin is pink in a white fetus; purplish in a black. Eyebrows and eyelashes are now present. There is fine, downlike hair all over the baby; the skin is rather wrinkled. At this point he or she is about 8½ inches long, weighing 180 grams (6 ounces). During these middle months the growth is substantial: by the end of the sixth month (27 weeks), the fetus will be 14 inches long, weighing 2 pounds, and starting to look very much like a real baby. If the baby were born anytime during this time, he or she might try to breathe, but would not survive.

"Something May Go Wrong!" and Other Anxieties and Fears

The many highs you experience in these middle months may be interrupted by a number of common fears and anxieties. Some manifest themselves in undisguised, nagging worries; others are expressed more subtly through dreams, the meaning of which may or may not be clear to you. These worries are on the narrow line between "psychological" and "physical," but because they most often relate to concerns about the child being normal, healthy, and alone (as opposed to being accompanied by an identical or nonidentical sibling;, this discussion is included in the "Physical" section.

"There were so many times during those months," Sally, a mother of a 3-week-old daughter noted, "that I just wanted to be held. I wanted him to make me feel secure and to help me brush all the worries I had away."

"I do a great deal of medical research," a science editor told me. "When I was pregnant I couldn't even go near books that had pictures of deformed babies. I'd shut my eyes as I turned those pages, read what I had to for my work, and slam the book closed."

"I worried about every imaginable thing," another new mother recalled. "About having a mongoloid or giving birth to a child with seven fingers or none at all; having twins or triplets or more; about getting cancer in the process. As soon as the baby started kicking I would panic if I thought it wasn't kicking hard enough or often enough. One night I dreamed I had given birth to a baby girl who had bunches of red carrots on her head instead of hair. She had pimples and eyeglasses and when the nurse brought her to me, I screamed, 'I don't want her!' " She laughed, looking down at her perfect, blond-haired, three-month-old daughter. "I guess vegetables were the theme of my worry those months because another night I dreamed I had the same baby, but this time it had white cauliflower hair."

Margaret Mead, in her autobiography, *Blackberry Winter*, writes of some of her anxieties of pregnancy: "During these months I had all the familiar apprehensions about what the baby would be like. There was some deafness in my family, and there had been a child who suffered from mongolism and a child with some severe form of cerebral palsy. There also were members of my family whom I did not find attractive or endearing, and I knew that my child might take after them. . . . What I dreaded most, I think, was dullness. However, I could do something about anxieties by . . . disciplining myself not to expect the child to be any special kind of person . . . of my own devising. I felt deeply—as I still feel—that this is the most important point about bringing into the world a child that will have its own unique and clear identity."

One woman reported to me: "I had this recurrent dream of giving birth to triplets, one white, one black, one oriental—and all speaking different languages. I didn't know where they came from, or who the father was." Lamented another, "I dreamt that one morning the newspaper carried a headline saying that eating apples caused birth defects. And I'd been eating dozens of apples for the past few months."

"I frequently dreamed of giving birth and then coming home with no baby," a middle-aged woman recalled. "I'd wake up in a cold sweat and touch my stomach to make sure it was there and still kicking." She then offered a description of a particularly unsettling dream: "I dreamt that when my baby was born I put her in a bassinet but it turned out later to be a coffin with the same frills and lace. You known I was never able to put any of my children in anything but a big sturdy crib where I would be sure to see all of the baby and make sure it was still breathing."

Not all dreams are upsetting, of course. Some, for example, might mix past and future to offer what you may feel is some insight about the unborn baby. "I dreamt that I was in a living room on a bright sunny day and my father, who had been dead for fifteen years, was there playing with my son whom he was calling 'Jimmy.' I woke up and told my husband, 'We're going to have a son named Jimmy.' And, indeed, that's what we did call him!"

Given the enormous physical and emotional upheaval of pregnancy and the fact that you are carrying a child whose characteristics and personality are now unknown to you, it is not surprising that there are anxieties and that some of these are expressed in dreams. But, again, some statistical observations and medical facts should offer some comfort: The overwhelming odds are that your child is normal and will be so at birth and after.

Genetic Problems and Amniocentesis

If, for example, you are worried about mongolism, technically known as Down's syndrome, be aware that under age 30, the odds of giving birth to a mongoloid child are about 1 in 1500; the chances are about 1 in 750 births and 1 in 280 births at ages 30 to 34, and 35 to 39 respectively; and between 1 in 130 and 1 in 100 at age 40.

If you are under age 35 and have no medical history to suggest that this genetic problem might occur, then you probably will have to learn to cope on your own with any anxiety you may have about mongolism, reminding yourself regularly that you are not in a high risk group. For you, amniocentesis—the procedure whereby a bit of fluid is removed from the amniotic cavity—is probably not a possibility. It is a procedure that is complicated and carries at least some small risk of its own. Since few medical laboratories are equipped to perform the fluid analysis, and your odds of carrying an affected child are so relatively low, your physician will probably not recommend it, and may discourage you from seeking someone to perform it.

But if you are over 35 and pregnant with either a first or later child, your fears about mongolism may have more basis. As the middle months of pregnancy begin, you will want to evaluate carefully the question of whether or not to undergo amniocentesis.

Amniocentesis is generally performed between the twelfth and sixteenth weeks of pregnancy. After a local anesthetic is administered, a needle is inserted into the uterine cavity and a bit of fluid removed. The procedure may, when you get results indicating "everything okay," relieve your concerns about mongolism or other genetic defects. But, as one 37-year-old woman related, the anxiety induced by amniocentesis cannot be overlooked either:

"We had waited a number of years to have a child; then it took two years to conceive. It all added up to me being an 'elderly primipara,' as the M.D.s love to call me. I decided I'd definitely have amniocentesis. But I really didn't understand the full emotional impact of that decision.

"I was beginning my fourth month when I had the test. It was a painless procedure and I was told that the risk to the baby was probably less than 1 in 2,000 because it was being done so early. What they *didn't* tell me beforehand was that I had to wait weeks— weeks!—for the results!" She spoke with emphasis, a bit of disbelief in her voice. "I was simply anxious for the first month. Then I fully panicked. I began calling the doctor every day, and all he could tell me was that the lab results weren't in yet. So then I began calling the lab—twice a day." She stopped talking to reflect on those trying and very long days. "You know, the really scary thing was that as I was waiting for the results, I was getting more and more attached to this growing life inside me. 'So what if it is mongoloid, I'll keep him,' I even thought more than once.

"I remember the day I got the results saying everything was all right even better than I remember the day I learned I was pregnant. For me, it was much more significant. I called my husband right away. It was like a ton of bricks had been lifted off our shoulders. The doctor asked if I wanted him to tell me the sex of the child. I said emphatically, 'No!' We had a healthy child and that was all I needed to know."

All the discussion about the benefits and availability of amniocentesis has to some extent obscured the fact that it is not a simple, quick means of diagnosis. The scientific method for prenatal diagnosis leaves much room for improvement. Certainly if you are at high risk of having a baby with any type of genetic disorder, have the test. But if you are not, don't insist that your physician refer you to a specialist to have it done. If you do undergo amniocentesis, the weeks of waiting will understandably be tense, but the advantage is that when reassuring news results, the remaining months of pregnancy should be almost worry-free.

Multiple Births

Probably no woman passes through the middle months of pregnancy without convincing herself that there is "more than one" baby in there. Again, you are dealing with greatly stacked odds against the possibility: one in about 88 pregnancies results in twins; the approximate square of that, 1 in 7,500, for triplets. (There is no truth to the rumor that because of unsettled events around the world, babies are increasingly hesitant to come into the world alone.)

Unless you have a family history of multiple births or have been taking Clomid (which somewhat increases the odds on twinning) or fertility drugs (which substantially increase the probability of multiple births), don't worry. Or perhaps it is not a worry, but a secret hope! If it does happen, it isn't necessarily a disaster!

Obstetrically, however, the interest might be more than a matter of curiosity in that if there are two or more babies, the approach at delivery may be different—so if there is a real concern that you are carrying more than one, your physician may suggest a sonogram (from "sonar," or sound navigation and ranging, reflecting its naval derivation). This "sound X-ray" uses very low energies and has no harmful effects on the fetus. Basically it will give you a "picture" revealing the size, position, and number of the fetus (or fetuses).

But even this procedure is not without some anxieties, as one woman related. "I was huge; we were all convinced that it was twins. My husband and I were panicked about the possibility, since we were still a bit uncertain about whether or not we wanted *one* child! I went over to the hospital and they hooked up their various wires to my abdomen. What they do is call out letter-number combinations to spot a point they want to examine with the machine—you know, like locating a point on the road map—D–12. Well, wouldn't you know in my case the first letter-number combination they called out was 'R–3.' And, of course, I thought they said, 'There *are three.'* I screamed. Then they told me that there 'are one.' "

Real Concerns

Some things are still worth worrying about during the middle months. Bleeding at this stage of pregnancy is never a healthy sign and, if it occurs, you should report it to your physician immediately. It may turn out to be no cause for alarm, but it is something he or she should know about.

Smoking, excessive use of alcohol, drug use, are still serious problems. Reread those parts of Chapter 2 if you are still not convinced! Eating a moderate, varied diet is essential, including a good amount of high-in-roughage foods to combat the constipation which frequently occurs in mid- and late pregnancy. (Again, see the appropriate section of Chapter 2 if you need a review.) Equally essential are regular prenatal visits to your physician, which include, among other things, check of blood pressure, weight, and urine.

Sex during the Middle Months

Masters and Johnson, and others who have studied sexual activity during pregnancy, all almost uniformly report that the middle months are a "sexual high," with sexual interest and activity not only improving substantially over the first trimester of pregnancy, but possibly surpassing prepregnancy interest as well.

Elisabeth Bing and Libby Colman write in *Making Love During Pregnancy:* "There are so many factors influencing the ups and downs of sexual interest and love-making during the course of pregnancy that general patterns that result from statistical studies are often irrelevant to the experience of one particular couple [but] the second trimester is generally the most comfortable period of pregnancy for making love. The initial adjustment to the idea of pregnancy has generally been made; if there were bouts of nausea or fatigue, they have generally passed. The chance of miscarriage is virtually gone. The abdomen may be starting to bulge but it is generally not yet large enough to present much of an obstacle to love-making."

Of course these comments do go under the heading of "generally." Sometimes nausea does persist. There may still be some fatigue or fears about miscarriage. Or you may experience some vaginal discomfort, although most women experience less discomfort because of the extra lubrication that comes with the genital engorgement of pregnancy. You may feel that with your abdomen puffing out like a souffle you are not attractive and your husband won't be interested. (As one woman described it, "I'm beginning to feel like I have a Supreme Court figure—no appeal.") Don't assume that he won't be pleased by your temporarily enlarged state. He might find the pregnant you to be very sexually attractive. On the other hand, the reality is that some men are indeed unnerved, a few put off, by a swelling abdomen. "I didn't know how to approach her," one expectant father sheepishly admitted. "I was afraid I might hurt her if I squeezed her too tightly. But more than that, I like my women slim. I wasn't turned off by her body, but it didn't turn me on either. I can't imagine what it's going to be like when she's really big either. I simply consider it a stage we have to get through to have the baby we very much want."

There can be no rules set forth on how to enjoy sex during the middle months, but perhaps there are guidelines. First and foremost, communicate with each other. Talk about the anxieties that may be inhibiting your sexual relationship. Don't, as often happens, ignore the subject, assuming that your partner, for whatever reason, just isn't interested. Second, particularly in the middle and later months of pregnancy, remember that "sexual pleasuring" need not always include intercourse. Experiment and adapt your techniques as your body grows and sex begins to appear logistically difficult. Third, if you're having difficulties, or have questions about sex during pregnancy, seek help. A good starting place is a book like *Making Love During Pregnancy*. Alternatively, raise the topic with your doctor.

Decision Making:
What Type of Labor and Delivery Do You Want?

I have always been absolutely fascinated with the idea of having a baby. When I was a teenager I used to be enthralled by the "Tell Me, Doctor" column each month in Ladies' Home Journal. *I loved to read about how the cells implanted and how the baby grew but the part I liked best was the birth. I've always been curious about what it would be like for me, how I'd react when labor began. I guess I'll find out soon.*

> —Jean, 24, high school teacher, ninth
> month

I have never liked anything to do with doctors of medicine—needles, hospital smells, the sight of blood all terrify me. Since I've been pregnant I've avoided everything possible on the subject of childbirth. I run the other way when I see a book on childbirth in a bookstore. I turn the television off if they are discussing birth. My doctor suggested I deal with my fears by going to Lamaze classes. I sat through one of them, but then they showed a film of a birth and I had to leave. I've talked to friends who have recently had babies, almost begging them to tell me it wasn't all that bad.

> —Susan, 22, secretary, eighth month

I figure that there will be some discomfort involved. I've often thought about what it would be like. When I had pleuresy a few years ago I was in a great deal of pain but kept telling myself, "You better get used to this; childbirth will be worse." I've had the same thoughts when I've had severe menstrual cramps. I am a bit worried, but I'll survive. When I see women on the street with children I often say to myself, "See, she survived it, and she did and . . ."

> —Ann, 25, housewife, sixth month

Would you believe, I never really thought about labor and delivery? I figured that billions of women before me had done it and survived. What's the point of worrying? I want a baby and this is what must happen. My feeling is that giving birth is a natural process; you don't have to learn to do it. It will happen, with or without my help. I have other things to worry about right now—getting ready for the baby, finishing up my assignments at work so I can take some time off. Labor and delivery are the furthest things from my mind.

—Barbara, 31, stockbroker, 8½ months
pregnant

During months four to six you will most likely make some decisions, or continue to reevaluate ones you have already made, about what type of labor and delivery you will have. Occasionally the decisions you make now are irreversible. (For example, some hospitals require that a husband must begin a preparation course at the end of his wife's sixth month if he is to be welcome in the delivery room.) But most often they are decisions left in a state of flux, subject to modification as your feelings change or you receive new information.

Frequently the prospect of making a decision about whether or not to enroll in childbirth classes, start exercise programs, learn about the physiology of labor and delivery, have the father present and participating during and after the birth raise anxieties and self-doubts and may bring about some conflicts between you and your husband.

Here we are going to examine some of the attitudes the two of you may have toward the processes of labor and birth, look at the reality of the pain and discomfort that may accompany childbirth, how you might cope with it, and, finally, how you might go about sorting out all this information to decide what method is best for you. Two points are immediately relevant here: First, there is no one right way to have a baby. You are not a better mother if you choose, for example, to avoid pain relievers of all types. He is not necessarily going to be a terrible father if he balks at joining you in the delivery room. Keep open-minded and flexible in making decisions on labor and childbirth. What is right for some couples is often wrong for you.

Second, instead of making the distinction between "natural childbirth" and "medicated childbirth," consider another dichotomy: *"prepared" versus "unprepared" childbirth.*

Natural childbirth to some may mean either drugless delivery, husband present, Lamaze classes, or some other combination of factors. It has to be one of the most "in" terms today. And the controversy about alternatives in labor and childbirth have become quite emotional, often based on the premise that the American medical "system" is out to rip off the pregnant woman, treating her as if she were ill and totally helpless, leading her to believe that birth is naturally risky, painful, and terrifying, and assuming that she has no sense whatsoever. (Much of this feeling of anger and resentment is reflected in Suzanne Arms's book *The Immaculate Deception*.)

The discussion here assumes you will be delivering your baby in a hospital or some other medically equipped place. It will exclude all references to controversy and instead attempt to look rationally at what alternatives are available and what the pros and cons of each are. Ultimately this is a decision the two of you will have to make for yourselves, optimally with the guidance of an understanding and interested physician who takes the time to offer assistance, if you need it, in decision making.

Attitudes about Labor and Delivery

The four expectant mothers quoted at the opening of this section express the gamut of feelings about labor and childbirth, ranging from the "Why think about it?" or "I'm curious" attitudes to ones characterized by mild or marked fear and anxiety. This latter end of the spectrum is worthy of some discussion because uneasiness about labor and delivery not only can be disquieting for the prospective mother and father during pregnancy, but also can heighten pain during the labor and delivery as well—turning what should be an exhilarating, rewarding experience into a long-dreaded, ultimately uncomfortable one.

From a historical vantage point it is understandable why women—and their husbands—feared childbirth. Until relatively recently the birth process was probably the most dangerous time in a woman's life. Indeed, Victorian women figured they had only a 50/50 chance of surviving childbirth and donned shrouds when the first labor pain was felt.

The message that "birth is painful" comes from many different sources. The Old Testament (Genesis 3:16) tells us, "Unto the woman he said, I will greatly multiply thy sorrow and thy conception; in sorrow thou shall bring forth children" (although there is still controversy among biblical experts as to whether the words "in sorrow" ought not to be translated "in hard work"). Euripides in 480 B.C. wrote: "Three battles are not equal to the pangs of one childbirth."

Classic literature is full of examples of painful, life-threatening labors. Kitty Levin's labor in *Anna Karenina* was so bad she probably wished that Adam had died with all his ribs. She is described as "flushed," "agonized," and "the terrible screams followed each other quickly until they seemed to reach the utmost limit of horror." Princess Lisa in *War and Peace* dies in childbirth following a "terrible shriek." In *Tom Jones* we are drawn a grim picture of Mrs. Fitzpatrick having a baby: "I became a mother by the man I scorned, hated and detested. I went through all the agonies and miseries of lying in . . . in a desert or rather, indeed, a scene of riot and revel, without a friend, without a companion, which often alleviate and perhaps sometimes more than compensate the sufferings of our sex at that time."

Of course we cannot overlook the obvious: These passages from literature were written by men (Tolstoy, Fielding). Women authors of previous centuries, either because they themselves did not have children or felt that the topic was too delicate to write about, generally ignored the subject.[1] In Jane Austen's novels, babies just arrive. Similarly, Charlotte Bronte in *Jane Eyre* omits any account of Jane's pregnancy and labor; the child just appears being placed on her father's knee. Pregnancy guides today, generally written by male obstetricians, also ignore the subject of pain, sticking to the strict clinical facts with which the writers apparently feel more comfortable.

Fear of childbirth—at least some fear—is probably more common than not. Dr. Helene Deutsch's comment that "Death always lurks

1. An exception here was Isadora Duncan, who herself must have had a rather unpleasant labor and childbirth experience. In her book *My Life,* she wrote: "Talk about the Spanish Inquisition! No woman who has borne a child would have to fear it. It must have been a mild sport in comparison. Relentless, cruel, knowing no release, no pity, this terrible unseen genie had me in his grip and was, in continued spasms, tearing my bones and sinews apart."

in the mind during birth" is somewhat extreme today, but worries about both your own survival and that of the baby are not at all unusual.

No one can predict in advance what your labor and delivery experience will be like. Some women—very, very few—even when delivering their firstborn, report a generally painless experience without benefit of any medication. It is far more likely that there *will* be some discomfort, certainly not the type described in nineteenth-century novels, but pain nonetheless. (Margaret Mead described labor as "pains one could follow with one's mind; they were like fine electric needles outlining one's pelvis.") During labor and delivery you will be vulnerable, dependent, challenged to keep control of yourself and the things happening to your baby. You will need the help of others, whether those others include your husband, a physician, nurse, nurse-midwife, and/or friend.

It is difficult here to attempt to discuss the pain and discomfort of labor and birth for a reader who may already have concerns. The purpose is not to exaggerate those anxieties, but rather to acknowledge that pain can, and usually does, occur, and to put the experience in some perspective.

Sandra, a 33-year-old designer who had recently given birth, had some comments which are relevant here:

"One of my now pregnant friends recently asked me, 'Was it really bad? How much pain was there?' And at the beginning I was hesitant to talk with her about it. I went through a natural childbirth class, entered labor as prepared as one could be, fully convinced that for me the whole thing would be a snap. Well, it wasn't. I was in labor for fourteen long hours, and because I thought I was going to be in total control, and because the conculsion that many of us in the Lamaze class reached was that the pain is all in your mind, within our ability to control, I was very unsettled when the powerful labor pains began. It turns out that I was nowhere near as prepared as I thought I was and felt defeated when I accepted the epidural offered me. I feel that if I had known that the pain at times can be intense, the element of surprise wouldn't have been there. And I've explained that to my friend, telling her that to me labor pains were like cramps in neon. Sometimes they can almost seem to overwhelm you. But they usually don't. There are a lot of different types of pain in life; many, many of them worse than those of labor. If you ask women who had long, hard hours of labor if they would do it again, most all would tell you yes. If it was really all that bad, I doubt that they would wish such misery upon themselves a second time."

Jennifer, 27, also offered her counsel about labor and delivery to expectant mothers: "I always intended to have a pain reliever—an epidural—during labor. My doctor and I discussed this briefly. What really came as a surprise to me was how late in labor I actually got the medication. Somehow I had in my mind that I had a choice of a medicated vs. not-medicated childbirth; one without pain, one with it. So the discomfort I felt until I was dilated enough to have the anesthesiologist called in was totally unexpected. If I had known about it, it probably wouldn't have been so bad at all. But I thought I'd just get a shot and never feel anything."

Linda Matthews, in *The Balancing Act,* had a somewhat similar comment: "Compared to what I had expected it was a shock. I had the idea, partly from our Lamaze classes and partly from my own ego, that my mind and body were going to lift me above the experiences of most women, that my delivery would be intense, but not overwhelming, and that I would always easily be in control. Well, it was intense—in a way I wasn't prepared for."

These experiences related by Jennifer, Sandra, and Linda have something in common. *All felt the discomfort they had experienced was intensified by the fact that they simply weren't expecting it.*

Relieving, Reducing Discomfort

Prior to the middle of the nineteenth century, there was no choice for women other than to bear whatever pain might accompany the delivery of their children. Then in 1853 Queen Victoria, in a controversial move, chose chloroform to make the birth of her seventh child more comfortable—despite the claims that by doing so she and other women were "robbing God of the deep earnest cries for help." After that, medicated pain relief during labor and delivery became more widely accepted and condoned, although there was—and still is—concern expressed about the possible undesirable side effects for both mother and child.

The description here of a few of the alternatives for relieving pain of childbirth is neither meant to be comprehensive nor designed to favor medicated over nonmedicated birth. However, while the notion of so-called natural childbirth is widely endorsed today by expectant and new mothers and a variety of health professionals, and may indeed be a marvelous experience for some couples, it must also be noted that, according to a number of obstetricians I consulted, a substantial number of pregnant women are totally uninterested in the prospect of labor and childbirth without some medication.

As comedienne Joan Rivers put it: "If natural childbirth, why not natural dentistry, natural appendectomies?" Another woman who had no desire whatsoever to find out what labor and childbirth are "naturally" like explained her viewpoint in a *Mademoiselle* interview: "To me there was nothing beautiful or appealing or interesting about childbirth. My part of the country—Texas—may have something to do with my attitude. In the South and Southwest there's no Puritan tradition, no conviction that you get anything out of going through something uncomfortable if you don't have to. You're much more inclined to pamper yourself."

While there is always a risk of taking any type of drug—and the rule "the less medication, the better" applies here—it is clear that if you have feelings like the ones expressed above, small amounts of analgesics or anesthetics when administered by competent medical personnel do not pose significant risks to you or the child. Furthermore, in many cases, the risks involved *without* such drugs greatly exceed the risks of using them. Again, the decision relative to the use of medication during labor and childbirth is an individual one, to be made by you and your doctor, without concern for what the latest book or women's magazine article said about what is "best."

Options

Only rarely today—generally in cases where complications are anticipated—are women put "out" completely during childbirth. Even fifteen years ago this was not the case. Widely used then was what was known as "twilight sleep," resulting from a combination of morphine and scopolamine, the latter an amnesiac or memory eraser and a member of the belladonna family.

It is not always easy to get an accurate recollection from women on whom these drugs have been used. The description offered me by one 45-year-old mother of three was typical of others of her age group: "I went into the hospital about three hours after labor began. I had decided very early in the pregnancy that going natural was not my style. The few girls I heard about who did were whipped, really worn out. Anyway, my doctor was there, gave me a shot, and I slowly drifted out. I must have thrashed around a great deal because when I woke up I had black and blue marks all over my feet and ankles. I realized that my baby was born because I was in a new room. Actually, I knew for sure when I saw the color of the sheets had changed. The labor room had blue sheets; there were white ones in the second bed I was in. I didn't even have to look at my stomach to know."

To many of us today this experience seems completely foreign. Serious health problems often resulted from the use of drugs like scopolamine: Babies developed respiratory problems or were born temporarily "doped up"; women under its influence often thrashed around violently, thus explaining the bruises that the woman above mentioned. Because of this and because more and more women are demanding to be awake and alert during their babies births, less scopolamine is used today, and more interest is demonstrated in local means of pain reduction. "Why be knocked out?" one woman asked of me. "You don't want to be knocked out the day you're married or on your wedding night—these are all big events in a woman's life."

Medication

Ask your physician to describe the alternatives to you. Be specific in your questions. Ask how and when during labor the drug is administered. (Don't, for example, assume, as Jennifer described earlier, that if you are going to have some type of pain relief it will be given as soon as you go into the hospital—it usually isn't.) Find out what the possible side effects are for you and the baby. The list he will recite will include forms of *analgesia* such as Demerol, or regional *anesthetics* injected into your body at a specific site, blocking off pain.

The *epidural* block, injected between two vertebrae in the lower back to cause numbness from the naval to the mid-thigh, is probably the most efficient and is being used increasingly—although it, like any other childbirth pain reliever, is not without limitations or risks. Since the epidural can lessen your ability to push and may slow down dilation of the cervix, it is usually not given until labor is well advanced. Use of an epidural also increases your chances of needing forceps at delivery and may have a depressing effect on your blood pressure.

Other regional drugs anesthetize the pelvis and are given just before birth or prior to the episiotomy (the incision to enlarge the vaginal opening, done in most deliveries to preserve the proper functioning of pelvic tissue). A *paracervical block*, injected in either side of the cervix and lower lateral borders of the uterus, will make the cervix and upper vagina completely insensitive. These and other medications used in labor and delivery are carefully supervised by an anesthesiologist or the physician, but even so, most do cross the placenta and some can make the infant drowsy, if only temporarily.

Psychoprophylaxis

Obviously, medication of any type is not always a necessity for successful, emotionally rewarding childbirth. Indeed, as mentioned above, some feel that drug-free deliveries are superior in this respect.

Dr. Grantly Dick-Read[2] set forth his ideas on relieving anxiety and pain in a number of books (*Childbirth Without Fear, Natural Childbirth Primer,* and *Introduction to Motherhood*). He maintained that childbirth is an essentially normal, physiological process and that most of the pain stems from poor conditioning brought about by the influence of old wives' tales and distorted reports about what labor was really like. The conclusion he drew was that fear in some way was the main agent for producing pain in labor. Fear, he wrote, overstimulated the sympathetic nervous system, leading to excessive muscle tone which in turn compressed nerve endings and

2. Dr. Dick-Read was a bit of a controversial man. His obituary carried in a 1959 issue of the *British Journal of Obstetrics and Gynecology* called him "a crusader with almost too much fire in his belly."

thereby caused pain. It became a vicious circle. Fear caused pain; pain increased fear. Eliminate the fear, Dick-Read suggested, and you will reduce pain in childbirth—without the use of drugs.

French physician Dr. Fernand Lamaze, drawing on the work of Russian researcher Ivan Pavlov—who had categorized a reflex as an automatic response of the body to some specific stimulus—expanded the Dick-Read theory, eventually, in the minds of many, totally replacing it. According to the Lamaze theory, when pain is perceived, there are other simultaneous sensations, specifically what you see, hear, or touch. By concentrating intently on one of the other stimuli, he suggested, pain may be diminished instead of occupying central importance.

The bases of the Lamaze method of psychoprophylaxis during childbirth include, first, a thorough understanding of the physiology of labor and childbirth to alleviate unnecessary tension and apprehension which only serve to enhance whatever pain might occur; second, muscle relaxation and training your body to deal with stress; third, development of a strong sense of concentration on another activity, namely breathing; fourth, learning through a series of training sessions to cope with stress with the aid of a coach, preferably the father of the child.

Elisabeth Bing, now considered one of the country's leading authorities in the area of prepared childbirth, detailed the use of psychoprophylactic pain relief in her book *Six Practical Lessons for an Easier Childbirth*, writing in much the same style as she addresses her weekly classes for expectant couples. She explains: "You will learn to change your breathing deliberately during labor, adjusting it to the changing characteristics of the uterine contractions. This will demand an enormous concentrated effort on your part. Not a concentration on pain, but a concentration on your own activity in synchronizing your respiration to the signals that you receive from the uterus. This strenuous activity will create a new center of concentration in the brain, thereby causing painful sensations during labor to become peripheral, to reduce their intensity."

Any discussion of the Lamaze or any prepared childbirth method, even a brief one like this, is incomplete without stressing the husband's role in the prenatal exercises, labor, and delivery. Indeed many new fathers have enthusiastically told me how this type of participation highlighted their own individual pregnancy experiences. "I couldn't recommend it more," one new father exclaimed. "I was hesitant at first. Somehow I thought I was going to be the only man in the class. Of course I wasn't. You get caught up in the spirit right away. It was an experience I would never have wanted to miss." "At the last moment my wife had to have a C-section," another new father explained, "so I didn't attend the birth. But all that preparation made me feel part of it anyway. I was there during most of the labor—and I really felt like I was doing something to help. I wasn't just standing around as an observer."

Husbands, Labor, and Delivery

Until very recently few obstetricians or hospitals would support couples who wished to be together just prior to and during their child's birth, whether or not they had taken courses in preparation for childbirth. (There are a few reports in hospital records of fathers being so determined to see the birth of their children that they handcuffed themselves to their wives as they were being wheeled into the delivery room.)

The traditional image of husbands in the hospital has been one of a man nervously pacing a waiting room, surrounded by coffee cups and cigarette butts, jumping up every time a nurse or doctor passed through the door.[3] His presence was often considered unnecessary, as an incident described in a 1950s magazine illustrates: A young naval officer on leave of absence with his pregnant wife requested an extended furlough so that he could be with her at the delivery of their first child. In response to his request he received a telegram which read: "U.S. Navy recognizes necessity for your presence at laying of keel. Considers your presence superfluous at launching."

Prior to 1970, a typical reaction of physicians to husbands' attendance at the birth was, as English obstetrician J. D. Flew wrote in a 1965 issue of the medical journal *Practitioner*: "Husbands should be

---

3. In earlier days, men apparently didn't wait in a hospital or simply pace outside the bedroom door. Henry Fielding's novel *Amelia*, published in 1776, describes what was a common practice: the expectant father holding a confinement party, with liquor flowing freely, and sending a bit upstairs every once in a while to his laboring wife.

in easy reach by telephone. . . . To me, the idea of the husband being present during [the birth] is repellant. It would put off my stroke and I would find it difficult to imagine any romance between this couple in the future." Dr. Joseph Rheingold, in his book *The Fear of Being a Woman,* concurs, adding: "Mature women do not wish their husbands to attend the delivery." And dozens of women who had children ten or more years ago went along with the opinions of these men, opinions which were probably the same as those of their own obstetricians. As one 44-year-old mother of three put it, "Trying to imagine Bill in the delivery room is like trying to imagine myself jumping into a volcano—too awful to consider beyond the first two seconds."

As with our approach to medication during labor and birth, our general attitudes have changed dramatically about having husbands present through labor and delivery and thereby allowing them to come as close as they can physically to experiencing the birth of their children. A growing number of couples today opt for making all aspects of childbirth a joint experience. If you feel strongly about your husband being there—and today most women seem to—tell him. But if he is hesitant, attempt to understand his feelings, too. For a variety of reasons, some men do have a fear of childbirth and simply do not want to witness it. You might simply ask a squeamish husband to keep the question under consideration, or suggest he speak with other men who have decided to be present at their children's birth (their enthusiasm may capture his interest).

Attending childbirth classes may help. As Elisabeth Bing told me, "Pregnancy can be the first real challenge a couple faces together in marriage. Talking about it, learning about pregnancy and birth can help. In each class a few expectant fathers admit that they have been 'dragged' over. But it is a rare husband who's been through the course, and then the hard work of labor, who doesn't decide that he wants to go in with his wife." If you are lucky, you may be going to a hospital which allows husbands to keep their options open: They can wait in the lobby, entering the labor room if they choose to; and if they decide not to be present at the birth, they may be given the option of watching the procedures through glass outside the delivery room.

Labor and Delivery: Making the Decision

Perhaps all the discussion in recent years about various childbirth techniques, and the benefits and risks of each, has served to exaggerate the importance of the style a couple chooses for the birth of their child. "The pleasure I see in having a baby was not the experience of it being born," one woman told me, "but in taking care of it afterward. Labor and delivery, relatively speaking, take a very short period of time. Why the big deal about it?"

Don't overstate the importance of these events to the point where you set unrealistic goals and possibly build yourselves up for the possibility of self-designated failure. If you see prepared, unmedicated childbirth as a challenge, one which you at least want to try to conquer, fine. ("Drugs just aren't my style. I've never used novocaine or anything like that. I want to see what my body is capable of.") If your attitude is that you will just wait and see what happens, how you feel at the time, and make a decision about medication then, that's fine too. ("I told my doctor I'd give it a try. But we agreed that he'd arrange for an epidural if it became too much for me.") And if you decide ahead of time, in conjunction with your physician, that you want some form of medication as soon as it can be safely administered, that's all right too ("I figure this is the age of modern medicine. Why not take advantage of everything they've got, as long as the risk is minimal?")

No one of these approaches is better than the other. But whichever you choose, some preparation for childbirth—for both of you—will most likely make the process easier and more satisfying. For you, the preparation may mean attending classes given at the hospital where you will deliver, at a maternity center in your area, at a Red Cross chapter or a church near you, or through an individual childbirth educator. (For example, in many cities child birth educators offer a series of six sessions, starting in the sixth month of pregnancy, for a total cost per couple of about $60.) Or the preparation may simply involve reading and studying books, and asking questions of your doctor or midwife.

Bring to whatever decision you make a sense of open-mindedness and flexibility. Childbirth, as any major life event, can be accompanied by unpredictable events and a little bit—or a lot—of confusion. Despite all the plans you make, you may in the end have to have a Caesarian delivery. Even if you think you want to avoid medication, a complication may occur which necessitates some type of pain killer. Or you may find at the last minute that your labor must be artificially induced—or assisted—by means of a drug such as Pitocin, a preparation which causes the uterus to contract strongly or on a more regular pattern. You can prepare and choose among options, but ultimately you must acknowledge that there may well be some unknown factors to be dealt with as they present themselves.

CHAPTER 5

"The Gentle Art of Infanticipating"

(Months 7, 8, and 9)

THE PSYCHOLOGICAL

The Final Miles of the Pregnancy Trip

Radiant. Uncomfortable. Anxious. Excited. Proud. Feminine. Frustrated. Fulfilled. Exhausted. Conspicuous. Optimistic. Impatient. Increasingly impatient.

These and other words describe the psychological experiences of months seven, eight, and nine of your pregnancy. The reality of your condition is now undeniable, inescapable. Any major ambivalences the two of you had are likely to be resolved, but you have some new, and a few of the old, worries to deal with. You will have the highs and lows, feeling pleasure at the imminent prospect of a baby, but also greatly sobered by the burden of the stark reality of caring for this unknown, dependent, demanding person. You are future-oriented, suddenly interested in catalogs of nursery furniture and baby clothes, but with a nagging uneasiness about buying things for someone who has not yet entered the world.

Anxieties, Worries

One night when Mary was in her eighth month, I was riding home on a bus and a father and his daughter—she was about a year old—got on and sat next to me. I'm sure that in my lifetime hundreds of parents and children sat next to me before, but this was the first time I really paid attention. Suddenly parenthood seemed very real to me—and, I might add, very exciting. But I wondered also if I had what it takes. "Maybe I should read more books about fatherhood," I thought.

—Harry, 23, graduate student

I had more than my share of morbid thoughts. I don't mean the normal things like worrying about a deformed child. I mean worrying about planes crashing and automobile accidents. I was a nervous wreck about the way my husband drove, although I basically consider him a good driver. He went on a business trip when I was in my seventh month and I had convinced myself within hours after he left

*that I was a widow and began wondering how I was possibly going to
raise this child myself.*

—Amy, 34, housewife, 8 months
pregnant

*Sometimes I feel very motherly. But what worries me is that at other
times I definitely don't. We were visiting with friends last week and
their kids really got on my nerves. I was so thankful to get back to the
peace and quiet of our apartment. Then I thought, "Oh, my God,
that's what this place will be like soon!" I hope I have a real surge of
maternal feeling when the baby is born—I'm counting on it!*

—Ellen, 29, fashion designer, 9 months
pregnant

Anxieties—about accidents, the possibility of tragedy ("I check
compulsively to see if he is still kicking"), your ability to parent effec-
tively, what the child will be like—are common in the last trimester
of pregnancy, just as they were in the first two. Each day brings you
closer to the acceptance of the reality of becoming a parent, with all
its responsibilities and privileges. Most men and women need a full
nine months to make the complete adjustment.

Particularly in the seventh through ninth months, expectant fathers make considerable progress in the transition to parenthood.
Even if he has been enthusiastic all along, your husband (as Harry
mentioned above) is likely not to feel the full reality of having a child
until during these months, and then only gradually. If he has been
hesitant and, in your mind, not as enthusiastic as you would like,
you will probably note a change for the better now.

(There are some very rare situations where ambivalence continues beyond this point. One woman I spoke with reported that her
husband argued with her in the taxi on the way to the hospital, saying he didn't want a child and suggesting they put it up for adoption.
The moment he saw his child was his time for transition—a sudden,
explosive one—to sincere, radiating enthusiasm.)

While you may have begun thinking of the image of your child a
few months earlier, it's possible that only now is your husband getting specific in his thoughts and anticipations. For example, up until

this time, he may automatically assume that the child will be a boy. A soliloquy in *Carousel* captures that feeling very well: A prospective father sings of the joys of his child, which he assumes will be the "spittin' image of his dad," but then stops short in sudden awareness that he had never thought about the other possibility. "What if he is a girl? What would I do with her? You can have fun with a son, but you've got to be a father to a girl."

Unusual dreams, expressing both worries and hopes, are common for expectant mothers and fathers at this time. "There were always at least two babies in my dreams," a new father (of one) reported, "and they all seemed to be different ages." "I was working on my doctoral dissertation just before I had the baby," a new Ph.D. explained, "and a few times in the last month I dreamed I gave birth to a string of letters."

In the last three months, psychoanalysts claim, women frequently have dreams involving falling, slipping, climbing through narrow places. Psychological researchers of all persuasions agree that dreams of babies appearing without the labor or birth processes are common, and usually these babies are chubby, attractive, six-month-old children, not newborns.

The anxieties may understandably upset you. The dreams may do the same or may simply be a source of interest or amusement to you. Either way you may derive some comfort from learning that they are normal, even characteristic, of the last trimester.

"I Was Square and Looked Like a Refrigerator Approaching"

That was how Jean Kerr, the humorist, described her last months of pregnancy (she was carrying twins). You may not necessarily feel quite that big, but given the tremendous growth of the fetus during this time, your self-image and your image in the minds of others will change dramatically.

You may be absolutely incredulous about how large you are, maybe even concerned about it, or you could be surprised that you're not larger, wondering, "How can a full-sized baby possibly fit in there?"

"I was simply enormous," one now very thin lady lamented. "I spent a great deal of time planning my diet for afterward—oh, and I avoided full-length mirrors too. That helped!"

"Was I ever huge!" another woman exclaimed. "There were a few times toward the end that every time I got into an elevator I thought, 'I hope it's planning on going down anyway.' Of course I knew why I was so big. It wasn't just the baby; I couldn't stop eating. I had this type of weird rationale: I figured that since I was going to have to go on a strict diet after the baby was born to get back in shape, I might as well eat up everything that was fattening now so I wouldn't be tempted later."

"When I was in my early months," recalled Emily, a woman who described herself as being due "yesterday," "I would look in amazement at women in my doctor's waiting room who were eight and nine months pregnant. I could hardly believe that I would actually get that large. I still don't think I am that big, but maybe it's just that now I have a new perspective."

"When I was in the middle of my eighth month I still thought I was fairly small for that state," June, a new mother, told me, "until one day on the street a group of young boys passed me, giggling and pointing to me. One said, 'Muy grande, muy grande.' I don't know much Spanish, but I knew what *that* meant!"

"I don't think there is anything more beautiful than a woman in her eighth or ninth month," wistfully declared a mother of three young children, one aged four and twins aged two. "I felt terrific in those late months. I liked being a big woman and despite the bulge in front still felt graceful. I think pregnancy was becoming to me."

"I looked terrible," another, just home from the maternity ward, exclaimed, appearing not terribly concerned about it. "I usually weigh 110 pounds. I was—well, let's say I was a hundred and plenty." She stopped and laughed. "I tried to go on a diet, but all I lost was my temper! My hair was always frizzed, my face was blotchy. I was physically ugly. But I didn't care how I looked to the world. I felt beautiful inside."

"What annoys me," Allison, in her eighth month, confided, "is that I have so little to wear. I bought a few basic maternity clothes, but could supplement them with a few of my loose blouses and sweaters—that is, until last month. Now I am down to my Basic

Six—a pair of slacks, a skirt, a jumper, and three blouses. My husband's shirts won't even button on me anymore. I think some new clothes would cheer me up immensely, but I'm darned if I'm going to spend money on things I'll only be wearing for a few more weeks."

"It might sound a bit contradictory and strange," a new father began, "but during those months I felt both proud and guilty. I was proud that I had been able to get Susan pregnant. I guess it's a type of macho thing that we all have. But I felt guilty that she who is so petite and frail was carrying this tremendous load and was obviously straining as a result of it. I kept asking, 'Are you okay? Are you okay?' about twenty times a day. I wanted to help her more, but I didn't know how."

No matter what your body image at this point, chances are you are having at least some trouble doing the things you normally do. Getting pots and pans out of a bottom shelf can be a major feat, requiring that you get down on your hands and knees in a position that will immediately stimulate those around to scream urgently, "Let me help you!" You'll discover, to your dismay, that department stores have a rather limited number of chairs for weary shoppers, and that, although you were previously unaware of it, your neighborhood suffers from a severe shortage of ladies' rooms.

As Others See You

As it becomes increasingly obvious that you are going to have a baby, you will find that people treat you differently. You are now definitely in the category of The Pregnant Woman and people have special reactions for you.

Some, especially those who have not seen a pregnant woman in a while, may instantly react to your size: "My goodness, you're getting big!" "You'll *never* make it until . . . (fill in your own due date)." "I've never seen anyone so large!" "There must be at least twins!" These are among the many comments you may receive, making you feel more "different" and conspicuous than you do already. Part of this may be just expected behavior of those observing very pregnant women, probably enhanced by the fact that the birth rate these days *is* at an all-time low, resulting in your being even more conspicuous and leaving others with a dearth of women with whom to compare you.

You may actually frighten, or at least unsettle, some others—especially if you're doing something outside their image of what a pregnant woman should do, like carrying packages, dancing, running, or reaching. (You will be told by at least one person, usually an elderly woman, that reaching will cause the umbilical cord to strangle the baby. Tell her that you really don't think that is true "anymore"!) Even if you are behaving "as you're supposed to," you may find people stand-offish. Dozens of women complained to me that taxi drivers wouldn't pick them up, that people avoided sitting next to them on trains and buses.

"When I was approaching my eighth month I had to make an emergency business trip by plane," one very pregnant accountant told me. "The stewardess greeted me as if I were smuggling a getaway car, asking, 'When are you due—this afternoon?' and then went on to explain to me how her airline was in the business of delivering people to their destination, not delivering babies. That really made me feel self-conscious." She stopped and then spoke with a bit of humor and sarcasm. "Just before the plane took off, the pilot looked out of the cockpit and I thought he was going to ask me to switch seats to balance the plane."[1]

Adrienne Rich, in *Of Women Born,* reports her personal experience of how pregnancy can make others uncomfortable. She had been invited to give a poetry reading at an old and famous boys' prep school in New England. When the headmaster found out she was seven months pregnant, he rescinded the invitation, explaining that it would be impossible for the boys to listen to the poetry, given

1. Most airlines do require that you have a note of approval from your physician if you plan to fly in your eighth and ninth months. You can understand their concern. A few years ago a woman in her eighth month went into labor on an El Al flight from London to Vienna (where she was going to see a specialist about some complications she was experiencing). She was delivered by one of the pursers whose one and only credential in the area of obstetrics was that he had delivered calves on a kibbutz in Israel. On arrival, baby and mother were in excellent condition, but it was not the type of incident El Al or any other airline would like to encourage.

the obviousness of her condition. This incident took place back in 1955, but some similar ones undoubtedly still occur today.

"I work mainly with men," a public relations account executive told me, "and when I was in my ninth month I was asked to give a speech at a sales conference in the town where I lived. I accepted, figuring there was no reason to tell the man who invited me that I was pregnant. Well, I arrived at the meeting and was astounded to find a room full of nervous, uncomfortable men who were tripping over each other to offer me a seat, though I preferred to stand. I had the distinct feeling that everyone wanted that meeting over—fast."

While you are in your late stages of pregnancy, many complete strangers will pat you on the abdomen "for good luck." If you were in a nonpregnant state they would never think of touching you, but now your abdomen is considered public property. Some will venture a prediction of the child's sex: "Now, *that's* a boy!" or "Let me see your nails; if they're flat it will be a . . ." or "Gee, you're carrying on your hips so it's a . . ." or "You're so high, that's definitely . . ."[2]

You'll find that sometimes out of the blue you'll be given advice: "I was in the elevator one morning on the way to work," one woman commented, "thinking about the activities I had planned that day, when a middle-aged woman started a sentence completely out of context: 'And do you know my daughter-in-law's doctor told her she probably couldn't breast feed. Can you imagine that?' I guess she thought that was exactly what was on my mind at the time."

Occasionally your condition may prompt casual observers to tell you in even more detail than before about their labor and delivery experiences. Or they may even relate some gruesome, pregnancy-related story, like how a friend's sister had to be delivered in an

2. Careful statistical analysis of these observations confirms that they are right about half the time. There is no way short of amniocentesis or X-ray to determine the child's sex. Heartbeat, position, or any other external indicator doesn't reveal what has to be one of Mother Nature's best-kept secrets. There was a doctor once who claimed he could predict the sex by the fourth month. He would never tell the prospective mother his prediction but explained he would register it in a big black book he kept and she could verify after the birth that he was right. Only after the physician's death was it discovered that he had two big black books.

emergency by means of a butcher knife, or something equally and unnecessarily frightening.

You may be pleased at the way people react to you during the last trimester—for example, when a stranger comes up and enthusiastically says, "Very soon! Very soon!" You may appreciate the extra attention that you get—possibly a seat on a subway or bus offered by a kindly gentleman or by a woman who remembers when she was in your state. (Don't count on such gestures. A number of women reported that they got no such courtesy, one indicating that when she was starting her ninth month and was forced to take a bus, a man sat there winking at her while she held onto the strap for two dear lives.) If you live in a large anonymous city you may feel particularly safe, for as one woman put it, "No one would dare attack or hurt you when you're pregnant. You're sacred."

The comments you receive from strangers, of course, are not always kind. There are always a few disturbed people who make obscene comments to pregnant women, or a few others who for some reason feel they must tell you "not to be ashamed" of your condition. "I wasn't surprised," a new mother told me, "that teen-age boys used to tease me or sometimes make me the object of their jokes, but what did surprise me once was when a middle-aged man, in a three-piece suit and carrying an attaché case, passed me and whispered, 'Hiya, preggie.'"

The public image of "expectant mother-person" may unsettle you. "What I disliked most," a 32-year-old receptionist informed me, "was that men other than my husband didn't find me attractive. I like being whistled at and flirted with. And all that stopped. Here I was, feeling quite sexy myself, but no one could see that. The men at my office kind of backed off, treated me differently. My image had definitely changed in their minds."

"I simply hated being conspicuous!" complained a new mother. "You know, the way some people stare at pregnant women, you'd think they still believe in the stork! I didn't like standing on a street corner, seeing a little boy point to me while his mother explained to him why I was in the condition I was in. I'm too private a person to be the subject of a sex education lesson." This same woman added another interesting observation: "When I was out in crowds or on the street, I found myself being very defensive. If someone's arm brushed by my abdomen I'd jump away. I was constantly trying to protect that area of my body."

The Ninth Month Is the Longest

At least it will probably seem that way. By the time you reach the beginning of your ninth month, or thirty-sixth week of pregnancy, you will undoubtedly have also reached the conclusion that you are terminally pregnant, receiving no consolation from those who remind you that the elephant's gestation period is six hundred days.

Once the final month begins, you start your countdown. "I even got my old calendar out and started recalculating," one mother related as she laughed. "I kept hoping I'd find out I was off by a few days and the due date was actually sooner."

"I don't count the remaining days in time," another told me, "but in events. I calculate now that I have 5 shampoos, 12 more times I have to master the feat of getting into bed without collapsing it, 12 more nights of insomnia due to flailing limbs, and 5 more trips to the OB."

Time is a burden for you now. You may try to make plans to fill the hours but discover it is difficult, given the frequent trips to the obstetrician—and the bathroom. The final days, which involve what Walter Winchell once called "the gentle art of infanticipating," will be made even more vivid to you by what can only be called the "Haven't you had the baby yet?" syndrome. "All month it happened," a new mother told me as she shook her head in resignation. "The nurses at the doctor's office, the mailman, the newspaper delivery boy, my parents, his parents, our friends, asking, 'Goodness! Haven't you had that baby yet???' It seems like the whole world had ceased operations, all waiting for me to 'do something.' "

"I learned a tip for the future," a woman in her ninth month revealed. "Always tell people you are due much later than you really are. My due date was yesterday, and the phone never stopped ringing. Every time I would try to take a nap someone would call and say, 'Doesn't your baby know that it's his birthday?' My father came over for dinner and accused me of being pregnant for twelve months!" Another new mother, listening to this one's complaints, interrupted. "It was worse for me. I was so huge that everyone in my family was convinced I'd be earlier. So the telephone calls started in my eighth month!"

"Frankly, it's getting boring," Alice, seven days overdue, admitted. "I think I would enjoy pregnancy more if it were only seven months. That's about my limit. I cleared my whole month's social and business calendar. And I literally have nothing to do. A month ago I was up to my knees in lists—not that I could see my knees! But now everything is done. The nursery is set, my suitcase is packed, and I'm just waiting. And it's as frustrating as looking for days at a nicely wrapped package which says 'Do not open 'til Christmas.' "

If nausea, anxiety, and food cravings are characteristic of the earlier months of pregnancy, the "phenomenon" often expected for the ninth month is something known as the "nesting syndrome." It may or may not happen to you. Some women report a sudden surge of interest in cleaning up their homes. "I got up in the middle of the night, took all the silverware and china out of the breakfront and scrubbed until dawn," was the way one woman described a symptom of her nesting syndrome, adding that she went into labor that next morning. "I found a huge stack of dinner napkins which I never had time to iron—and I ironed nonstop until they were done" was a "symptom" reported by another. It's difficult to say if there is such a thing as a nesting syndrome in humans, or whether it is an attempt either to fill in the hours of waiting or a matter of pure practicality, preparing for the expected infant.

What can you do to make the ninth month seem shorter—or at least to get the most out of the waiting period? Some advice offered by recently pregnant women:

"Above all, rest! You need a supply of energy for the first days of motherhood. Take advantage of the free time! You may not be able to sleep so well ever again!" "If you have a job and are physically able, consider working right up to the last minute. Just go about your regular routine, and keep your eyes off the calendar." "Get out—enjoy yourself. Go out to dinner, because two weeks from now you'll probably need a baby-sitter, that is, if you even feel like going out then." "Call your most immediate friends and relatives and update them on your condition, guaranteeing that you'll let them know 'as soon as something happens' and then take your phone off the hook." "Get a few good books, get into bed or a comfortable chair and read." "See a few movies or shows. Get out and live as if you only have a few days of life left. Because in a sense . . ." "Take short walks and lots of deep breaths. It helps calm you." "If you have the energy, make a few frozen dinners so that you don't have to cook for the first week or so after you get home from the hospital." And, above all, "Try to relax!"

THE PHYSICAL

By the time you begin your seventh month, your baby weighs about 2 pounds and is some 14 inches long. The hair on his head is developing, his eyes are open, and the skin still has a wrinkled appearance. By the beginning of his eighth month, the length is 16 inches and the weight just under 4 pounds. Although each day approaching your due date increases the child's chances of survival, a child born alive in this month already has over a 50 percent chance of survival. (The age-old superstition that a baby born in the seventh month is in some way superior to, or has a better chance of survival than, an eight-month baby is hogwash. It is merely based on the superstition of many primitive peoples that the number seven, because it is the number of phases in the moon, is a lucky number.)

By the end of the eighth month the weight will have reached over 5 pounds, the length over 18 inches. Gradually the skin becomes smooth, although it is still covered by a cheeselike secretion. The wrinkled look disappears and a layer of fat develops under the skin. During the last four weeks of pregnancy the baby is capable of gaining one-half pound a week. By the end of the ninth month the volume of your uterus has expanded 500 times and its weight has gone from under an ounce and a half to 30 ounces.

Discomforts of Late Pregnancy

What else can be said except that it is no surprise that such rapid growth and the sheer weight you will be carrying around inside you has got to lead to some discomfort.

For example, "heartburn" (which has nothing to do with either a burn or the heart) is a classic discomfort of late pregnancy. Any internal profile of your pregnant self would reveal why: The upward displacement and compression of the stomach by the enlarged uterus, and decreased gastrointestinal action, causes the stomach to empty more slowly. Basically, you are suffering from the type of indigestion that overweight individuals often experience. But, at least in your case, it is temporary. Try a tablespoon of cream a half-hour before meals. Ask your physician to recommend an over-the-counter type antacid and, obviously, avoid foods that cause pain. (One woman told me that throughout her pregnancy she craved cucumbers topped with creamy cucumber dressing. And although a huge serving left her practically moaning with pain, the taste was so rewarding she concluded it was worth it.)

Given that your uterus is exerting tremendous pressure on your bladder, you find that you have to urinate more frequently, even when your bladder is not very full. Constipation may continue to bother you since your entire intestinal tract is not working very efficiently. Make sure you are getting sufficient amounts of fluid and roughage (coarse cereals and leafy vegetables, for example) and ask your physician to recommend a laxative or stool softener. Hemorrhoids can be a real bother, one which can cause problems later if not attended to. In the late months of pregnancy the veins at the rectal opening become enlarged. Hard bowel movements can cause the veins to protrude, causing local pain, bleeding, and itching. Effective remedies are available, but you should ask your doctor about them, not self-prescribe on the basis of an ad in a women's magazine. Similarly, if your problems include varicose veins, nosebleeds, and nasal congestion, leg cramps, swelling of the ankles, frequent urination, and backache, be assured that you are not the only pregnant woman to experience these discomforts, and that your doctor *has* heard of them before—and probably has a few means of dealing with them. As has been the case throughout pregnancy, some symptoms are not just discomforts but may signal trouble and necessitate an immediate call to your physician. Among these are bleeding, intense headache, high fever, dizziness or blurred vision, and puffiness of the hands and face.[3]

Sex after the Seventh Month?

Why not? You may find that your interest in sex is still very strong. Aided by a bit of imagination on the part of both you and

3. It is likely that your ankles and legs are puffy now. But it is swelling of the face and hands that is a greater source of concern. This type of swelling, in conjunction with elevated blood pressure and albumin in the urine, signals toxemia, a serious pregnancy disorder.

your husband, it can be as rewarding and enjoyable as ever.

If you are comfortable about having intercourse and your physician has not given you a specific reason why you should avoid it, there is no risk posed to the child. Many couples do still worry about the possibility of causing an infection in the baby by having coitus, but all studies in this area indicate the fear is unfounded. Sexual intercourse does *not* introduce an infection to the baby that is safely protected in an unbroken bag of fluid on the other side of a closed cervix. Female orgasm with the resulting contractions, in all but a few special cases, will not hurt the baby or bring on labor before you are ready.

Bing and Colman in *Making Love During Pregnancy* point out: "The resolution period of the sexual arousal cycle takes much longer during pregnancy than at other times. The uterus may stay hard for several minutes, particularly late in the pregnancy of a woman who has been pregnant before. . . . The normal increase in the blood flow to the genital area, which is typical of sexual arousal as well as pregnancy, causes feelings of fullness and swelling." The authors go on to point out that while it can be frustrating and uncomfortable in its advanced stages, sexual relations in the third trimester are often characterized by heightened sensitivity and more frequent orgasm in some women. Can orgasm late in pregnancy initiate premature labor? Medical opinion is still mixed on this subject. Since it does cause the uterus to contract, a woman with a particularly sensitive uterus or a history of trouble carrying a baby to full term might be asked to avoid having an orgasm. But it is apparent from the Bing and Colman study and others that most women who enjoy both intercourse and orgasm to the very end of their pregnancy do so without complications.

Even though it is not medically contraindicated, however, a substantial number of couples do, beginning in their seventh month, have intercourse less frequently. "Quite honestly," a few women told me, "I wasn't eager to be flaunting my body. I just didn't think he'd be interested in having sex with the baby in the way."

"We never really talked specifically about it," one expectant mother told me. "We just kind of called a moratorium about then. I guess we were a bit worried about harming the baby, but moreover, I was always exhausted and, well, it got awkward."

"We simply became platonic friends," reported another. "We both made this decision without ever actually talking about it. We knew our sex life would resume afterwards, so neither of us was worried. I wasn't as frustrated as I thought I might be. He used to make jokes about how *he* was, but it was nothing for either of us to worry about."

"We stopped having intercourse," reported a number of other couples, "but we most definitely did not stop making love." This latter point is stressed repeatedly by the authors of *Making Love During Pregnancy*, who note that logistical difficulties or fear of harming the baby, if they cannot be resolved, should not lead to the total dissolution of the physical relationship at a time when a couple should feel closer to each other than they ever have before.

How Will I Know If It's Real Labor?

Don't worry. You will know. If birth is imminent the labor pains clearly announce themselves for what they are. But before we look briefly at the symptoms of true labor, it's worth pausing to look at the advice you will inevitably receive about "how to bring labor on" if you are approaching or beyond term.

Castor oil doesn't work! Neither does anything else except the medically oriented preparations meant for the purpose of inducing labor (which can be administered only by qualified medical personnel). And there is no reason to believe that you can either wish yourself into labor or prevent it through mind control, although Dr. Helene Deutsch does relate an interesting story on this subject:

She tells of a woman who, because of a family history of miscarriage, had a great fear of losing her baby. She found comfort in a friend who was also pregnant; the problem was that her friend was due a month before she was. This was a great source of anxiety to her—the fact that she would be "pregnant alone" for four full weeks. And her friend, sensing her worry, subsequently gave birth one month late—on the exact day her anxious friend became a mother! Deutsch claims she verified this report, adding that the ten-month gestation child's growth was more than equal to the normal growth of a child outside the uterus. She concludes: "Apparently, Mrs. Smith's friend had mobilized all the energies of the 'retaining powers' in order to help Mrs. Smith by waiting for her term." (One wonders if Mrs. Smith's friend could have held out if there were two months difference in the due dates!)

As a followup to this story, Dr. Deutsch tells us that Mrs. Smith decided, with her friend's psychological help, to get pregnant again. Both did the same month. But this time the friend packed up and moved away during the third month. (If you had a friend like this maybe you would too!) Mrs. Smith immediately miscarried.

How will you know if the labor is real?[4] At first you will have some doubts. It may begin as no more than a low backache, not dissimilar to that which you've probably experienced with increasing frequency during the last few weeks. But those dull pains then begin to creep around to the front. Unlike what are known as "Braxton-Hicks" contractions, the chief characteristic of true labor is its rhythmic nature, the recurrence of contractions at fixed intervals. As labor progresses, the interval from the beginning of one pain to the beginning of the next is gradually shortened from fifteen or twenty minutes, to three or four minutes when labor is well underway. Of course, even if this is your first pregnancy, you may be different. You may find that your first labor pains are immediately four to six minutes apart. This may not mean birth is imminent, but rather that it is your unique laboring "style."

True labor is often accompanied by a pinkish vaginal discharge ("the show") which is different from the whitish discharge you probably experienced during the last few weeks of pregnancy. Occasionally, women have labor announced with the sudden breaking of the bag of waters—the amniotic fluid. There are many descriptions of the early labor process in books on the biology of pregnancy. Here what is important is to set aside the anxiety that you won't know and will be caught in an elevator on the way to the hospital when you should be on the delivery table. It hardly ever happens to any woman in the U.S. today—and it's exceedingly rare for the primipara. ("First babies just don't 'pop out,' " was how one obstetrician summed it up.)

---

4. You'll find a more detailed description of labor in the next chapter.

Breast or Bottle?

Now is the time to start thinking about this important decision. It is not a matter of "seeing how you feel" after the delivery. Successful breast feeding requires preparation—possibly toughening up your nipples through daily scrubbings and other means to minimize chance of pain when you begin breast feeding (consult your physician about this), letting your OB know if you will be needing medication to stop milk production if you choose not to breast feed, and preparing yourself psychologically to feel comfortable with either alternative.

Be open-minded in evaluating the question. There is no one right or wrong answer here. Unfortunately, much like the issue of medicated versus nonmedicated childbirth, the issue of breast feeding has been surrounded by a number of emotional arguments which often lose sight of facts and personal circumstances. There are advantages and disadvantages of both. Consider all of them. Discuss them with your husband, doctor, and friends—and then decide.

What are the advantages of breast feeding? First, although the manufacturers of modern-day formulas have done an admirable job in attempting to simulate mother's milk, there is today no formula which exactly duplicates it. Formula often contains more than three times as much protein (which is not necessarily an advantage) and significantly less carbohydrate value than does mother's milk. Cow's milk is approximately four times higher in riboflavin content than is human milk. These and other differences explain why some infants, but certainly not all, have some difficulty digesting the formula, at least in the beginning.

Second, much can be said for the warm relationship breast feeding can foster between mother and infant. Many women appear to gain a great sense of fulfillment when they are able to breast feed successfully and they feel that the child benefits from the security of the close body contact.

Third, breast feeding may be less expensive than bottle feeding. Basic infant formula can cost about $6 or $7 for six quart-sized cans—which will last a week to a week and a half—plus the cost of bottles, nipples, and cleaning and sterilizing equipment.

Fourth, the act of sucking sends a reflex nervous impulse to the mother's pituitary gland. This in turn not only initiates the lactation process, but also causes the new mother's uterus to contract firmly, thus promoting the return of the uterus to its nonpregnant state.

Fifth, breast milk does contain antibodies, offering immunity to some viruses and bacteria.

And sixth, some studies suggest that breast feeding practically eliminates the possibility of overfeeding because the infant naturally stops when he is satisfied, whereas a bottle-feeding mother may feel compelled to get every ounce of the formula she has so carefully prepared from the bottle into the baby.

In fairness, however, these various benefits listed need some perspective: First, while infant formula isn't an exact match for mother's milk, it is a scientifically prepared product which has nourished millions of babies for many years.

Second, bottle feeding does not mean that you necessarily lose the physical closeness at feeding time. If you hold your baby in a position closely approximately that of breast feeding, it is possible that very little of that intimacy will be sacrificed.

Third, breast milk isn't exactly "free" either, since it requires greater consumption of food by the mother. It might be argued that the additional daily dollar value of $.60 to $1.00 here is comparable to the cost of buying prepared formula.

Fourth, there are drugs which are generally administered after delivery to speed the return of the uterus to its nonpregnancy condition.

Fifth, while breast milk does offer some forms of immunity, your baby will be born with a type of natural immunity that will protect him through the first few weeks. In an environment such as ours today in the U.S., where high levels of sanitation and immunization are maintained, exposure to harmful microbes is all but eliminated anyway. Thus this quality of human milk takes on less importance.

Sixth, while breast milk offers a built-in control mechanism, this does not mean that bottle-fed babies are doomed to become obese. If you choose to bottle feed, you can keep the overfeeding possibility in mind and correct for it. With very little effort on your part, you will quickly become attuned to your baby's indications of when he is satisfied.

Are there any benefits of bottle feeding? Although it is almost sacrilegious in today's back-to-nature world to admit it, the answer is definitely yes. Indeed, for years people as far back as the ancient Greeks have been searching for an adequate substitute for mother's milk. Until this century, wet nurses were common in aristocratic households. So awareness of the advantages is nothing new.

First, and most obvious, if you choose the bottle, you can get help in feeding. Your husband or someone else can take over when you want to sleep or pursue other activities. Husbands whose wives bottle feed are often enthusiastic about this opportunity to develop an intimate relationship with their children during feeding time, an opportunity of which they feel they would otherwise be deprived if the child were solely dependent on his or her mother. Second, for some women it is reassuring to know exactly how much milk the baby is taking. In breast feeding the amount consumed is an unknown. If you are feeding by bottle you can count ounces.

Third, for many, breast feeding offers the advantage of getting back to normal activities more quickly, resuming work, social events, and a regular sex life. (While some women report feeling a significant increase in sexual interest during the time they are breast feeding, others complain that their husbands are put off by their feeding, almost resentful, and that this is reflected in their relationship together.)

It is a matter of choice. Decide what is right for you. Maybe none of the advantages of breast feeding appeal to you, but you simply want to have the experience, to see what it is like, to "give it a try."[5] Or maybe you are personally convinced, without any list of pros and cons, that breast feeding is the best way to feed a newborn. If this is your decision, fine. But don't ridicule or deprecate others who choose to bottle feed. If you are leaning away from breast feeding, be assured that your infant will be well nourished on whatever formula he is given; and if there are problems of indigestion or constipation, a new formula can be tried. Bottle feeding is nothing you have to apologize for or feel guilty about. It does not mean you are less of a mother or less of a woman. In all aspects of pregnancy—labor, delivery, and parenting—make the decisions that are comfortable for you.

5. For further information you may want to write to the La Leche League International at 9616 Minneapolis Avenue, Franklin Park, Ill. 60131.

CHAPTER 6

Baby Coming!

(Labor and Delivery)

THE PSYCHOLOGICAL

This Is It!

The Real Thing

I had just seen the OB the day before, a few days before my due date, and his reaction was "Nothing much happening." So my husband and I settled down for a long wait.

The next morning I woke up at 4 feeling very hungry. I got up and made myself an orange juice and honey concoction, and with it wolfed down a large piece of chocolate cake. Then I went back to sleep. At 6 I woke up with some pretty strong contractions. So I got up and went into the bathroom and discovered that the "show" had appeared. I realized that this was the day I'd hoped for and dreaded for months.

Then suddenly I was very composed. I took a shower, washed my hair, shaved my legs and waddled into the bedroom. My husband was still in bed, with one eye open, but the moment he saw me fully dressed, suitcase in hand, he leaped out as if a fire alarm had been sounded.

He started timing my contractions. They were already about 10 minutes apart, so we decided to call the doctor. When I told him, "I think I'm in labor," his response was, "But you weren't anywhere near ripe yesterday!" I felt like a rejected peach!

We drove calmly over to the hospital and I was immediately ushered into this little room while my husband was sent down to fill in admitting papers. Sometimes I think they invent that job for the husband just to keep him occupied. Anyway, I'll never forget that examination room. It was so stark white, so clinical. They left me there for about 10 minutes, and I began to get a little bit frightened. Then a parade of medical students, interns, and residents came through to check me out. Next came the prep and enema—the less said about them, the better. Would you believe that I used to be modest about going to the gynecologist?

*I never planned to go the natural bit. So when I was finally taken
into my labor room I said, "Where's my shot?" I was a bit surprised
that I had to wait a few hours. Well, yes, I've got to say it was an uncomfortable few hours. But having my husband there—and eventually
having an epidural—made it bearable. Listen, at that point I was
about to give my doctor my rings as long as he stopped the pain. I
don't understand how a woman can do it alone, without someone who
cares, without a friend. The nurses and doctors are efficient, but they
are ice cold. They must know what you're going through, but they've
watched it so often they're removed from it. Once when a pain was really severe, I moaned, and I heard one of the nurses in the next room
say, "Oh, shut up."*

—Alice, 26-year-old high
school French teacher

*I had this creeping backache on Tuesday night, three days after my
due date. I called the doctor to describe it and he recommended that,
if I could, I try to relax and go to bed early, and call him in the morning. We both went to bed about 11. I woke up at 5 with some fairly intense pains, about seven minutes apart. A few minutes after that I felt
something warm and wet between my legs and knew my waters had
broken.*

*We held off until 7 and then called the doctor. He told us to meet him
at the hospital at 9:15. John and I had decided in advance that when
the time came we weren't going to tell anyone else that labor had
begun. We figured there was no point in putting other people—our
parents, for instance—through it. And we thought it was just too personal to share with anyone else just then. So we sat on the couch talking quietly to each other until it was time to go. We both fully realized
what a special day this was going to be, that before it was over, our
baby would be with us.*

*I'll always remember that when I put my coat on to leave I turned
back and stared at the living room and thought, "It will all be so different when I next return here. My whole life will be changed. This
house will never quite be the same again."*

*We'd both taken the Lamaze course so were prepared for what would
happen—prepared for almost everything. We planned basically to*

deliver our own baby, having the nurses and doctors do as little as possible. What annoyed us at first was that as soon as we got there they separated us. Don wasn't allowed to be present during the initial examination—and afterwards they kept asking him to leave the room each time they checked to see how dilated I was. I almost got angry but said to myself, "Look, Sarah, you're going to have a baby. Don is here. Don't rock the boat."

The pains did become intense, but with the breathing and the help from Don, I stayed on top of them. Beforehand my doctor had made it clear that there was an anesthesiologist on hand if I needed him, but I never really felt I did. The middle stages were the toughest. By the time I was starting to push, I was too excited to feel pain. When I look back on it, I was in labor quite a while—eleven hours after I got to the hospital. You know, when I think of driving a car nonstop for eleven hours, I'm exhausted at the prospect. But labor wasn't that bad. We had some pictures taken in the labor room. Between contractions I looked pretty good. It was Don who looked haggard.

The only thing I really had to complain about was that I felt my doctor let us down. His partner was on vacation and he had a full office, so he wasn't there when I needed him. When I began having the urge to push, he still wasn't there. I was put on "hold," told not to push, for his benefit. The next time, if there is one, I might consider a midwife, someone who might give me a little more personal medical attention and be there when needed.

> *—Sarah, 31-year-old investment banker*

I had some vague menstruallike cramps around 10 in the morning on my due date. I didn't quite know what to do right away. The one thing I dreaded was getting to the hospital with my suitcase and then being told to go home because it was too early. That happened to a girl friend of mine.

About noon I called my doctor and asked him what to do. He told me to come over to his office. That gave me hope that this was real labor, so my husband rushed home from work and we grabbed a cab, only to be told by the OB that it was "too early." He told us to go home and wait. Now that was frustrating. We were sitting around for four

*hours, just waiting and wondering. I simply couldn't get comfortable
no matter how I tried. I alternately paced around the living room,
watched television, and drank hot tea. We even tried a bit of Scrab-
ble. When it got to be six o'clock and my contractions were more
severe, Jim said, "Let's go. I don't care what the doctor says." I told
the nurse at the OB's office that we were on our way.*

*Despite my discomfort I had to laugh at people's reactions to us as
we left our place both times and tried to find a cab. There was no
doubt in anyone's mind where we were going! The people in the
elevator looked at me, white with fear. And when we finally found
cabbies they had looks of "why me?" on their faces.*

*We had planned on a fully drug-free delivery. Actually, we were
going to make a celebration out of it! We'd packed an iced bag of
shrimp cocktail and two splits of champagne in a picnic bag, and fully
intended to enjoy them as soon as we got out of the delivery room. But
things didn't exactly turn out that way. As soon as I was admitted,
labor all but stopped. I was given some Pitocin to speed things up
again. The contractions were intense, but I felt in control, and
thought things would proceed normally. Only then did I learn that I'd
have to have a C-section. I was given a local anesthetic and I did see
the birth of our child. I felt like I missed a great deal, not completing
labor and having a normal, regular birth. But it was Jim I felt badly
about. I know he felt cheated. He had so much looked forward to
being there at the birth, to holding his child as soon as it came into the
world. Oh—he ate the shrimp and drank his split of champagne at
home alone that night. I didn't exactly feel up to it.*

—Greta, 27-year-old housewife

The Moment of Birth

*I was wheeled out of the labor room down a long corridor. My hus-
band was right there. We just smiled at each other the whole way.
There was an atmosphere of excitement in the rooms we passed as one
nurse confidently announced, "Baby coming!" as we moved along.*

*Once I got in there, the baby came right away. What can I say except
it was the thrill of our lives. I don't think either of us yet has come
down from the high of that day. My only regret is that I forgot to take*

*my glasses into the delivery room and had to squint as I looked in the
mirror to watch the birth!*

> —*Janet, mother of a
> 3-month-old son*

*I had gone through the preparation, but I really didn't know how ex-
cited I would be. Frankly, I was also a bit nervous at the last moment.
It was so clinical-looking in the delivery room, I once thought, "What
am I doing in here?" A moment later I knew..I was fixated the moment
the head began to appear. I gasped to my wife, "He's here! He's here!"
A second later, I realized that "he" was a "she" and we all had a good
laugh. I feel that I really participated in my daughter's birth and it's
an experience I will never forget.*

> —*Thomas, 38-year-old attorney*

*Only a few billion people have had babies before, but this was very
special. This was ours. We have never felt closer together than we did
on that day. We laughed and cried when we first saw him. "Danny,
you're here. Welcome!" I said as soon as he was brought to me.*

> —*Terry, 24, mother of a
> 4-month-old son*

*I never was a religious person. I hardly ever go to church or anything
like that. But when I saw that perfect little baby emerge from my
body, all I could think was, "Thank you, God."*

*My husband wasn't in the delivery room, but he was watching
through a glass window in the door. I remember seeing a patch of
dark hair on her head as she began to appear and the doctor saying,
"It's a girl," loud enough so my husband could hear too. Then I asked
three times, "Is she all right?" The nurses kept answering, "Of course
she is!"*

> —*Martha, 22, housewife and mother*

*I will remember Ann's birth as being one of the most special days of
my life. But I recall being a bit unnerved by what I felt was a lack of
maternal feeling. When she was handed to me on the delivery table I
studied her for a long time, almost wondering, "Who is this little per-*

son whom I don't know, and where did she come from?" For me, the
maternal feeling and bonding came a few days later.

—*Sandra, 23, nursing student*

I don't think any man or woman who watches a birth ever forgets it.
It is an event I don't think any man should miss if he has the chance.
When I saw my son it was love at first sight. Of course I was ready to
throw him out the window four weeks later! But that moment was
very, very special.

—*Jack, 25-year-old insurance
salesman*

I didn't have the rush of feelings I expected. I'd say my immediate reaction was, "Well, there she is. So that's what I've been carrying all
these months." I was numb from the waist down so I didn't have too
much mobility. I sort of lay there staring at her. I realize now that
part of the reason I didn't have any really strong surge of emotion is
that I was simply exhausted. I'd been in labor eleven hours, and up
for twelve hours before that. I really just wanted to eat something
then go to sleep.

—*Mary, 33-year-old secretary*

I don't exactly know what I had in mind—I had never seen a newborn baby before. And I was a bit shaken when I saw mine. He looked
a little bit like a turkey—a long neck and lots of red, rough, dry skin. I
laugh at myself now—and my wife still teases me about "our turkey."
But at the time I was a bit worried.

—*Kevin, 25-year-old father
of a 3-month-old son*

For some reason my wife and I assumed our child—our
firstborn—was going to be a girl. We always referred to her during
pregnancy as "Cynthia." Now that I look back on it, I guess it was
because my wife so much wanted a daughter—I didn't care as long as
it was healthy—that she convinced both of us that's what it was going
to be. When I saw it was a boy I was taken aback at first, almost
feeling that while we gained a child, we'd also lost Cynthia.

—*Allan, 31-year-old radiologist*

Your Baby's Birthday: A Perspective

You will very likely remember vivid details of the day or night you begin labor, as well as all the events and circumstances surrounding the birth of your child.

You may well have a few "mental rehearsals" for the event, imagining well ahead of time what will happen and how you will react.

"I always imagined going into labor around 10 in the morning," one new mother recalled. "In my reverie I'd call my husband at work, leave a message with his secretary (who was very nervous, very excited when I calmly told her) that I was going to the hospital and that he should meet me there as soon as possible. He'd arrive around noon, the baby would be born at 4 and we'd have champagne and caviar at dinner time." (This same woman pointed out that things don't always work out the way you expect, noting that her labor began at midnight and her child was born at 9 that morning, and their celebration consisted of orange juice, cereal, and coffee.)

Whatever your labor and delivery experience, you may well go over and over in your mind the circumstances under which you got the message that "this is it" and the events of the hours that followed. It is well known that many men love to relive and tell of their war experiences, if they can find someone to listen. The same can often be said about mothers—new and old—although the analogy here is not appropriate in any other way.

What will be your reaction when you get an indication—be it "show," regular contractions, breaking of the "bag of waters"—that you are in labor? This is quite impossible to generalize about. If you are prepared in the ways of pregnancy, labor, and childbirth—as a result of reading or attending classes—you will likely be excited and more than a bit curious about what is going to happen in the next few hours.

Of course you'll continue to hear stories about expectant parents, particularly soon-to-be fathers, panicking the moment labor begins and remaining in that condition until after the birth. Classically, the will-be father is pictured putting on his clothes backward—that is, if he puts them on at all—as he rushes off to the hospital; being unable to get the car started and getting lost on the way; when he finally arrives, calling for a wheelchair and getting into it himself; and then pacing around the waiting room murmuring, "I hope it's a girl! I hope it's a girl so she won't have to go through this." *Expecting* magazine reports the story of a husband who was so nervous, so ruffled, that when he was told to slip on a sterilized, open-back hospital gown upon arrival in the labor room, he proceeded to take off all his clothes except his socks and sneakers.

You will react to labor and delivery in your own style. But it is very unlikely that you will fit any of these nervous stereotypes. On the other hand, no matter how prepared you are, how much in control of things you plan to be, keep in mind that even when everything goes well, labor is generally somewhat of a challenge and things often do go other than as you planned. Keep open-minded, remain flexible.

Such a highly personal, emotional, and imminently memorable moment as the one when your child is born cannot be described impersonally in the pages of a book. The couples quoted at the beginning of this chapter offer the only adequate description. You, when the day comes, will have your own individual and special reactions to add.

Most reactions are fully positive. But others, as the quotes indicate, can be mixed with a bit of guilt and self-doubt. It *is* one of the most exciting events of your joint lives. But don't build it up to the point that you are disappointed if bells don't ring and lights don't flash. And don't be disappointed if in the delivery room you don't feel a sudden surge of motherliness. In one sense, the transition to parenthood is a very sudden one. A few hours before you may have been watching television with your husband in your neat, peaceful apartment. Now, all of a sudden, you are being handed a screaming newborn. You may instantly feel a closeness, a warm maternal feeling, but then again, it could take some time.

THE PHYSICAL

When Labor Begins

Labor is the term given to the entire process of bringing your baby into the world. It is traditionally divided into three states: Stage 1 covers the period from the onset of labor to full dilation of the cervix. Stage 2 begins when the cervix is dilated and ends when the baby is born. Stage 3 is the delivery of the placenta.

Three out of every four babies are born within eleven days of the estimated due date. What starts labor? This has not been fully established, but it is now generally believed that hormones secreted by the infant himself, probably by the infant's pituitary gland, start the process.

As we noted in Chapter 5, different women have different types of labor onset. But there are usually three distinctive signs that labor is about to begin. The first is the onset of regular, strong uterine contractions, occurring every 15 to 20 minutes (although they may well start closer together than this) and lasting from about 30 seconds to a minute. They are uncomfortable, but not necessarily painful. When they occur you can feel your uterus contract and become hard. A second sign is the rupture of the bag of waters which lies in front of the baby's head and is held within the uterus by intact membranes. The rupture may occur suddenly, with one big gush, or the leakage may be slow. The fluid is clear and sweet-smelling. (One woman told me she thought it smells like laundry bleach.) A third sign is the passage of a small amount of blood-stained mucus called the "show." Other common signs of approaching labor (though not the actual onset) are diarrhea, backache, and decreased movement of the baby.

Once moderate and regular labor pains are felt, the show has appeared, and/or your waters have broken, you should contact your physician for further instructions. He may tell you to sit tight for a while longer, awaiting word from him or, depending on your symptoms, he may suggest meeting you at his office or the hospital within the hour. If you report any of these symptoms he will undoubtedly remind you not to eat or drink anything, since a recent meal may rule out the use of a general anesthesia (should it be needed) because of the possibility of vomiting which could lead to serious breathing problems. Some physicians allow clear liquids—but not including vodka! Don't drink milk, as gastric acid forms a solid from it.

Whether or not you plan to have any form of anesthetic it is important that you follow this rule. At this point you have no way of knowing if such medication might become necessary.

During the early part of labor your cervix slowly—or quickly— begins to open. Before labor begins the walls of the uterus are thin, the cervix long and thick. The situation now beings to change, the cervical canal becoming shorter. This process is known as effacement, measured in percentages from zero to 100 percent. Once your cervix is effaced, the force of the uterine contractions is devoted to dilating the cervix, that is, opening the mouth of the uterus. Full dilation is 10 centimeters (the latter a term you will be very familiar with by the time your baby is born).

Dilation is generally slow during the early part of labor. Once labor is really underway the contractions become stronger and closer together and the rate of dilation picks up.

Hospital Routines

Hospital routines vary so greatly it is difficult to generalize about them here, but most often your husband will be sent off to work on "papers" soon after you arrive. As Alice mentioned earlier, this often seems like "busy work" to keep him occupied while you have the initial examinations—especially given that so much of the paper work relating to insurance and admission are completed days or weeks before you get to the hospital. In any case, the separation is usually a short one, which must be endured.

You may initially be placed in an examination room where your vital signs (pulse, blood pressure, and temperature) are taken, your labor contractions timed, and the extent of cervical dilation evaluated. A "prep" of the pubic hair (usually partial, but sometimes complete) may or may not be done, depending both on your preference and standard hospital procedures. Most likely you will be given an enema, as the bowel is directly adjacent to the birth canal and emptying it provides as much room as possible for the passage of the baby. An enema also prevents you from expelling some feces as you bear down during delivery. If you are not feeling particularly terrific at this point anyway, the enema and general examination may make you feel nauseous and may lead to a short-lived bout of vomiting.

In most hospitals today you will also be monitored—both for baby's heart and for your uterine contractions. The monitor gives a continuous picture of the fetal environment. (Don't panic if the beep you hear is not always regular. Sometimes the monitor slips off your abdomen, or the machine is somehow defective.)

Once you are settled in labor room, your real work begins. And labor can be just that: plain, hard work. By the time you are six centimeters dilated, contractions may be very strong, possibly occurring every two minutes and lasting a full minute. Just as you are reaching eight centimeters, and lasting until the full ten, comes the hardest and shortest part of labor, known as the transition. Contractions may be two minutes apart, lasting from sixty to ninety seconds. The closer you get to this stage, the more intense will be the contractions. Then, suddenly, as you begin to feel you can't take any more, you will begin to feel another type of sensation—a pressure on your pelvis and an almost uncontrollable desire to push or bear down, although you will be told not to push unless you are fully dilated at that point. (If you've had an epidural you most likely will not have this urge to push and the nurse or doctor will instruct you here.) By the combined force of your pushing, and the exertion of the abdominal muscles and uterine contractions, the baby's head descends and stretches the pelvic floor, coming into contact with the perineum (the muscular outlet of the pelvis). At this point, to enlarge the opening, an episiotomy—incision of the perineum between the vagina and anus—may be performed. And your baby is ready to be born.

Born—With Help

Sometimes you know before you enter the hospital that because of the position of the baby, a previous operation you've had, or some anatomical difficulty, you are going to need some specialized obstetrical service—for example a Caesarean section.[1]

Statistics from around the country indicate that about one in every 15 to 18 births is done by C-section, although informal observation of delivery patterns in large cities like New York suggests that the percentage is very much higher than that, possibly being one out of every 8 or 10. The most common cause for a C-section is a previous Caesarean birth, but the decision to perform this operation may be the result of a narrow pelvis, large infant, unsatisfactory progress in labor, toxemia, or some other complication.

Basically, Caesarean section is the delivery of the fetus through a surgical incision in the uterine wall. A general or regional type of anesthesia may be used. Often the complication that makes the operation necessary will determine the choice of anesthesia.

If your baby's head fits your pelvis without any disproportion, your membranes have ruptured, the cervix is completely dilated, *and* there is still some type of problem—either the baby being in distress, a slowdown in labor, the head being higher than it should be, or something else—your physician may elect to use forceps, two separate thin steel blades with inner surfaces curved to fit the sides of the infant's head. The blades are inserted into the vagina to grasp the head and aid in extracting the baby. The use of forceps will require that there by some anesthesia used.

If you have long been planning what you anticipated would be a fully uncomplicated birth, it can come as quite a shock if a C-section must be performed, if forceps must be used, if the birth must be induced, labor speeded up, or if there is any other type of surgical intervention—perhaps caused by the baby being in a position which makes a spontaneous delivery difficult. No matter how much planning you do, you cannot eliminate the possibility that you may need

1. It has often been said that the operation received its name from Julius Caesar, who was born that way. This is very unlikely, given that the current level of medical technology would have led to his mother's death on the spot, and we know she lived for many years after that. More likely the procedure derived its name from the Roman Law of about 725 B.C., "Les Caesarae," which ordered that this operation be performed on any woman dying during the last few weeks of pregnancy, in order to save the child.

some sophisticated obstetrical aid in delivering your child. This should not be a reason to feel let down that you missed a truly "natural" childbirth. As we stressed in Chapter 4, to put so much emphasis on the birth itself is to overlook the full participation of the nine-month pregnancy experience—and the years of shared experiences you have ahead of you.

The Appearance of the Newborn

If you have been having dreams of what your baby will look like, you most likely have an image of a beautiful, bouncing, red-cheeked, six-month-old baby. In reality, newborn babies look a bit "funny" after they are born. Sir Winston Churchill once put it this way: "All babies look like me—bald, wrinkled, and frequently purple with a bad temper."

Concern about the baby's appearance can mar the birth experience and lead to unnecessary worry, so it's worth taking the time to emphasize that newborns are not handsome picture-book babies, bright, alert, and smiling. At birth their skin is covered with a greasy coating known as vernix (which is usually completely washed away during his or her first bath, in or near the delivery room), and with long hair known as lanugo (which characteristically disappears after a few weeks). Sometimes the skin has a slightly bluish tinge immediately after birth.

A newborn's head may have an unusual elongated shape (a condition which improves within a few days), and generally a baby's feet and legs look quite bowed. (This should be no surprise, given that he or she has had both feet tucked up near the head in rather cramped quarters for the previous few months.)

One of many concerns observers of newborns have is about apparent "anatomic asymmetries." Perhaps you will have someone ask you if your baby's mouth curves up (or down) on one side, if his dimples are crooked, if one testis is higher or lower, if one arm or leg moves more vigorously. You might wonder if your baby's breasts appear a bit puffy—not knowing that male newborns, having been exposed to the hormones in his mother's body, often exhibit this sign of breast stimulation.

Or the eyes may appear swollen, probably as a result of pressure on the eyelids when medication was dropped in after delivery. If forceps were used, there may be some slight marks on the skin of the face and head, but these fade away after several days, What is often mistaken as a "forcep mark" is a triangular pink area, which technically represents a collection of tiny capillary blood vessels close to the surface which are visible through the highly transparent skin of a baby. Popularly, these are known as "stork bites" because they also occur at the bottom of the neck, and in "the old days" were explained by noting that the mythical stork transported the baby to his waiting parents by grasping the infant's neck in its beak. The actual cause of this slight mark is not known, but what is known is that it disappears gradually over the first year or so of the infant's life, being pale at times, mildly red when the baby is crying hard.

So-called "mongolian spots" in the skin at the base of the spine, commonly seen in babies of Mediterranean heritage, are also a constant subject of inquiry by parents and sundry relatives. One mother I talked with insisted that this was a bruise which resulted from the baby's being spanked after birth. But she eventually accepted the fact that this was a natural type of pigmentation which would fade rapidly.

When you think of some of the serious problems which can affect infants (less than 2 percent of infants have anything even approaching a serious defect at birth), it is absurd that new parents and their relatives are anything but delighted at the birth of a perfect child. But if you do have some anxieties, ask your doctor about them. An assurance that your concern is both normal and unfounded will set your mind at ease. You can then fully appreciate the definition set forth by Irving S. Cobb: "A newborn," he explained, "is merely a small, noisy object, slightly fuzzy at one end, with no distinguishing marks to speak of except a mouth . . . but to its immediate family it is without question the most phenomenal, the most astonishing, the most absolutely unparalleled thing that has yet occurred in the entire history of this planet."

CHAPTER 7

After the Fact

THE PSYCHOLOGICAL

What is technically known as the "puerperium" (Latin for "having brought forth a child") begins the moment you give birth and continues for several weeks. From both the physical and psychological points of view, these weeks can be exciting, complicated, and generally tumultuous, although not necessarily negatively so. It is a time when your body is undergoing major changes en route back to its nonpregnant biological state. Indeed, at no other time in your life do your bodily tissues and your emotions change so drastically in a short period of time. It is often a time of emotional upheaval, perhaps characterized by your feeling very, very high—and at the same time, increasingly pensive and worried.

As with all major life transitions, there can be some rough going as you gradually develop a new self-confidence and begin to restore some order to your daily life and your relationship with those around you. Unlike the circumstances in days past where you would have been surrounded by dozens of relatives and/or servants during this period, you may instead feel very much alone.

Suddenly You're Someone's Mother

If you were now playing a word association game, your response to the card which reads "postpartum" would almost inevitably be "depression" or "blues."

It is unfortunate that the term postpartum immediately conjures up an image of a new mother in a frilly nightgown in a hospital maternity ward, surrounded by vases of flowers, candy, and baby gifts, and weeping miserably. Or the image of another young woman at home sobbing into a pillow as her distraught husband stands beside her, their infant in his arms, wondering what awful thing he said or did to trigger such a flood of tears.

True, some 40 to 60 percent of new mothers, and an unknown percentage of new fathers, report some feelings of depression. Hippocrates, the "Father of Medicine," commented on this phenomenon years ago,[1] and descriptions of hospital wards in earlier centuries often refer to bars on the maternity ward as a precaution against the allegedly unpredictable behavior of new mothers.

There *are* dramatic physical changes during and following the birth of your baby; for example, a 30 percent loss in blood volume, continued contractions of your uterus, shifting of the position of a few internal organs. But the after-baby blues could not be purely a physical phenomenon, a matter of biological destiny for all new mothers, because women who adopt babies also report the same symptoms—and many fathers, adopting or not, do too. The position taken here is that postpartum depression is not inevitable but is largely the result of external circumstances, and the fears and insecurities are of a nature that can be anticipated and dealt with. So instead of looking directly at the "postpartum depression phenomenon," we will examine some of the broader emotional issues you'll be facing once your child is born, ones which, if they are not well understood and controlled, could make you a victim of postpartum blues.

The Nonpregnant You

This is one change that happens very quickly. After nine months of getting accustomed to the pregnant you, you're a nonpregnant woman again, yet you don't really feel or look like your old self. Your emotional reaction to this new state may be either positive or negative—and most likely a little bit of both.

Suddenly you have a new and different body image. "I felt a type of void when the baby was born," one new mother told me, "like something very important to me was missing. I couldn't easily get used to the fact that the bulge wasn't there."

"I really missed having her inside me!" another woman laughingly confessed. "We were so close for such a long time, then suddenly she was in the nursery down the hall. That first night I really

1. Hippocrates had a somewhat confusing biological explanation for this form of depression, indicating that it was the result of suppressed lochia (the discharge from the vagina in the days following birth), and to a diversion of milk to the brain, complicated by a sudden influx of blood to the breasts.

longed for her. If I had it to do over again, I might find a hospital where I can have rooming-in."

"Not me!" her friend exclaimed. "I was so exhausted before the birth I felt I had given all I could inside me. It was time for him to grow on his own. I was delighted each time the nurse brought him for me to feed. But I must also say that I was happy when she came to take him away too. I just wanted some rest, to get my strength back."

These two women describe opposing feelings that, if they were candid, probably were detectable to some extent in both of them. You probably *do* in some ways miss the bulge. Such a feeling is very normal in the first days after birth. Cécile Sauvage, in one of her poems, aptly describes the feeling: "I am a hive whence the swarms have departed. He is born. I have lost my young beloved. . . . I am alone." Dr. Therese Benedek made a similar observation, expressed in more scientific lingo: "The trauma of birth interrupts the biological symbiosis between mother and infant."

On the other hand, you were probably getting a bit weary of lugging all that extra weight around and you are attracted to the idea of being able to move around relatively unencumbered once again. But you're still not yourself. You still feel big, ungainly, and certainly flabby in the middle. You're in an in-between state and probably feel more than a bit uncomfortable about your body image. The fact is that it will take some time for you to return to your prepregnancy size, shape, and weight. You are going to feel somewhat "dumpy" for a while, so don't make things worse by trying to force yourself into one of the sveltest dresses in your wardrobe. Pick a few transition garments, ones which are a bit loose and free-flowing. (Most women find that it *is* depressing to wear maternity clothes once the baby has arrived.)

Worries

If you really work at it, you'll find that there is an almost limitless list of things for you to worry about in the postpartum period. So right from the start, try to keep yours to a minimum.

The worries may start right after birth. "They told me in the delivery room that he was perfectly normal," Janet, a 34-year-old new mother told me, "but I guess I didn't believe them. I kept asking the nurse when I got back to my room, 'Are you sure everything is all right?' And when they first brought him to me, I immediately took off his clothes to make sure he had all his parts."

Concerns like this about "everything being all right" are very common in the first days of motherhood, and they can be aggravated by all those friendly, meddling people who come to see you in the hospital and during the first days you're home. "When my best friend came to the hospital," Alice, a 26-year-old mother of a 6-month-old daughter, exclaimed, "she walked in saying, 'Gee, I just went by the nursery. She looked awfully quiet. Hope everything is all right.' Then my aunt arrived gushing, 'Oh, she's simply beautiful, and I'm sure those forcep marks will go away eventually.' Then my mother came in telling me that she thought it was very strange that my daughter didn't open her eyes very often, and then added that she hoped my 'beer belly' would disappear soon and the color in my cheeks return. My goodness! They had me half hysterical!"

Why exactly visitors feel compelled to make comments of this type is a mystery, but it very frequently happens and if you take it to heart it can be one of the many factors contributing to depression. Ignore their comments and, as we discussed in the previous chapter, if you do have concerns, raise them with your obstetrician or pediatrician.

In addition to commentaries which suggest that the baby doesn't meet all the expectations of your friends and relatives, you, independently, may find that reality doesn't always jibe with expectations. "I had in mind this cooing, laughing baby—someone I could have fun with," another new mother explained. "So I was at first a bit let down when I was handed a sleeping infant who didn't seem to care whether I was there or not."

"It just wasn't what I expected," another new mother told me. "I don't know exactly what I *was* expecting, but it was different." Dr. Benedek points out that there is an emotional lag after parturition, resulting from the intense emotional buildup of motherliness during pregnancy, followed by the lack of it after the child is born, when the mother secretly asks herself, "Is this all there is?"

On your list of worries, if you have decided not to breast feed, may be the notion that you made the wrong decision. "When I was first handed my daughter," a brand new mother confided as I spoke with her in her hospital room, "and I saw how she instinctively turned to my breast, I felt suddenly guilty, very inadequate as a mother for not having at least tried to breast feed. I talked to my husband about it, and he admitted to me that he felt the same way, like we weren't doing everything to give the baby the best start in life." This feeling among non–breast-feeding mothers is very common, primarily because by that point the option to breast feed is no longer available (the mothers having been given medication to stop the flow of milk). The feeling is typical of any irreversible decision where both alternatives were attractive and generally disappears as suddenly as it appeared.

Your worries—which, if they get out of control can lead to depression—go beyond concerns about the baby itself. The reality is that the stereotyped picture of the joyful mother and her newborn does not begin to suggest the full range of feelings, positive and negative, you will experience. You may berate yourself, or just quietly feel guilty, if you don't have a surge of maternal feeling toward this bundle which is put into your arms four or five times a day. After all, it is a one-way street for a while. Babies don't respond to your love by offering theirs right away. Relax—for you, "motherliness" may take some time to develop. You may within days after the birth feel panic about what you interpret as total ineptitude in the practical art of mothering. "We both went to the Red Cross preparenthood classes, one woman lamented, "and I learned how to diaper a doll. Let me tell you, there is more to early motherhood than that!"

"I was so naive that I had to have the nurse show me how to put a disposable diaper on," another woman told me, laughing and noting that she subsequently learned that almost every new mother needs such lessons in basics. "And after I got home, the first time I found the crib sheet damp, I actually thought it was from tears!"

Your concerns may be related to the extreme vulnerability you see in your child. "Do you know what depressed me?" another new mother asked. "Right after I got home from the hospital I began dwelling on an event that occurred twenty years ago. When my mother was pregnant with my younger sister, my father had an affair with his secretary and my mother was so terribly hurt. I'll never forget how defeated, how devastated she was when she found out. I thought, 'What if that ever happens to my daughter?' I couldn't stand to ever have her hurt that way."

When you leave the hospital, the most common anxiety you are likely to experience is the one which might be termed the "is she still breathing" syndrome. Betty, a 30-year-old mother, described the symptoms of this classic phobia: "Each of the four nights we've had her home I've gotten up in the middle of the night, tiptoed in, and put my hand on her back to see if she's still alive. I know that must sound crazy, but the moment I wake up I'm seized with the fear that she has suffocated or something. Sometimes I have to press down so hard on her that I end up waking her up. But at least then she cries and that's proof she's still with us."

Betty continued, "Last night I woke up at four absolutely panic-stricken. I dreamed that we had fallen asleep with the baby in bed between us and that my husband had rolled over on top of her. Does this sound normal? And how long does it go on?"

It certainly is normal—and the breathing check may go on for months. Very, very rarely, unpredictable events such as "crib death"—even now a poorly understood phenomenon—can occur. But if you make sure that your child is fed, burped, clean, and safe in a crib (without pillows, very heavy blankets or quilts when he or she is very young), you have done all you can.

Mixed and Mixed-up Feelings

Ambivalence—about your separation from your child, and your general feelings about parenthood and the baby—is as common in the postpartum period as it was throughout pregnancy.

If occasionally, in the hospital and when you get home, you feel resentment toward this new, demanding creature, be aware that you are not alone in those feelings. Jane Lazarre, in *The Mother Knot*, expressed the reaction that every new mother must feel, if only transiently, in the first days and weeks of parenthood: "Who was this immensely powerful person, screaming unintelligibly, sucking my breast until I was in a state of fatigue the likes of which I had never known? Who was he and by what authority had he claimed the right to my life?"

"I pronounced myself a monster after two weeks," a new mother confided, with a smile on her face. "There were times that I got so frustrated when he cried that I wanted to shake him, while at the same time accusing myself of lacking all maternal feeling and wondering if I hadn't made a mistake by getting pregnant in the first place. A minute later I would ask myself, 'How could you feel this way toward this innocent, helpless thing?' Then I'd be depressed. My advice, based on experience, is, 'Don't be overly critical of your negative feelings. Just because you feel like stuffing him down the toilet, you shouldn't feel guilty about it.' "

Obviously, if you find yourself verging on physical violence to a young baby—or any child for that matter—you have a problem that may require professional help if it doesn't soon resolve itself. It's better to let the child cry with the door closed than to react impulsively. But the feelings we are discussing here are temporary thoughts of 'Why did I even have her?' or 'I simply can't take it anymore,' and the subsequent guilt feelings that inevitably follow. Those are normal; those will pass.

All the Little Things

The emotional shift from pregnant to parent may be exacerbated by little annoyances—chores that accumulate, slightly caustic remarks, just plain doubts about whether you can handle your new assignments and responsibilities, and sometimes, a very real sense of aloneness.

"I was really the center of attention late in pregnancy," another woman explained. "And during the labor and birth everyone was around encouraging me. But then my son was born, my husband went home to get some rest, and I was very alone in the hospital room. I really wanted someone to lean on myself then, but I realized that the support relationship I had with my obstetrician was terminated. I had a dream that night that I was nursing a woman—and the woman was me."

"I was super-excited the day we were supposed to leave the hospital to go home," a bright, smiling new mother recalled. "I was dressed about four hours before checkout time. The nurse gave us a bag of 'new-parent goodies,' a bottle of sugar water in case the baby cried on the way home, escorted us to the door—and then we were on our own. We were terrified on the way home. You know the way newlyweds put a 'Just Married' sign on their car? Well, at that point we wanted a 'Just Babied' sign so people would approach us with caution!

"Anyway," she continued, "we got home and put the baby in the bassinet. He cried and cried—and we just stood there helplessly looking at each other. We had never had a new baby before! What were we supposed to do? Even after he went to sleep we still thought we could hear him crying—we eventually called it the 'phantom crying syndrome.' We never seemed to be able to relax. The burden of responsibility at that time seemed overwhelming."

Unless you take steps to avoid it, when you get home the emotional crisis may intensify somewhat. From a practical point of view, there are probably chores to catch up on. The food supply may have dwindled, the laundry accumulated. The phone may be ringing incessantly with the greetings of well-wishers and would-be visitors. Little tasks may suddenly appear overwhelming. "I was trying to get dinner on that night, just a simple steak and salad," one mother of two remembered. "The baby was crying; my husband was frantic about what to do with him. Then all of a sudden I realized that we didn't have any prepared salad dressing in the house and that I'd have to make it from scratch. I just sat down and sobbed, 'It's all too much for me.' Before I had my second, I made sure there were five jars of salad dressing in the house!"

Overreaction to mild criticism or slightly caustic statements is not at all unusual in the postpartum days. If you are prepared for this possibility, perhaps you can laugh as the tears start flowing. "I was having some difficulty breast feeding—but I was determined," a mother of a week-old baby explained. "Yesterday my mother-in-law stopped by and, seeing my frustration, said, 'It's ridiculous to keep trying. You obviously have no milk.' I burst into tears and sobbed for an hour."

"When I got home from the hospital I called my mother—she has seven kids—to ask her advice about feeding the baby," a young mother of a two-month-old son told me. "She said, 'Give him a tiny bit of cereal right away, no matter what your doctor says.' I told my husband what she said and he exploded, saying, 'Leave your mother out of this!' I was so hurt I cried the whole afternoon."

"I was feeling very high when I got home," a 28-year-old career mother told me. "I was looking through the dozens of cards, flowers, and gifts people at work had sent, then all of a sudden I realized that one person I worked with hadn't sent anything. I was low for the rest of the afternoon. It was the emotions inside of me that wanted to cry, not the rest of me."

Avoiding Postpartum Depression

Can you avoid postpartum depression? Well, at least you can take some steps to minimize your risks.

First, don't assume that you will automatically develop the blues. There is no known physical basis for the phenomenon. It is not inevitable—you can fight it.

Second, *get help*. New babies demand an incredible amount of time, attention, and hard work. One woman I spoke with who had recently survived the first five weeks of her son's life told me it was so exhausting that she now regrets not having twins to get the rough parts in the lives of the two children they wanted over with all at once.

Daffy definitions of "a baby," culled from various sources, communicate an idea of what those early days will be all about. What is a baby? "A bald head and a pair of lungs"; "a tight little bundle of wailing and flannel"; "an inestimable blessing and bother"; "a perfect example of minority rule"; "a disturber of the peace"; "the most desirable pest"; "a curly dimpled lunatic"; "an alimentary canal with a loud voice on one end and no responsibility on the other."

Before you go into the hospital ask your husband or someone else to keep up with the housework and shopping so you don't return to a disaster scene. If at all possible, make arrangements for someone to help you for the first two or three weeks after you get home. A professional baby nurse can be ideal, but that isn't your only option. Ask your mother, mother-in-law, an aunt, sister—anyone who you feel is competent and interested and with whom you feel comfortable—if they could lend a hand. Don't feel that you are less of a parent if you can't do it all yourself. *More than any other factor, pure exhaustion may be the primary underlying factor in postpartum depression.* ("Where did that baby get all its energy?" one new mother exclaimed. "She left me walking into walls at the end of the day. I began to think I should be drinking that formula too. Maybe it would pep me up as much as it apparently does her.")

Joan Rivers, in her book *Having a Baby Can Be a Scream*, humorously describes the experiences she, her husband Edgar, and their new baby, Melissa, had in the early weeks: "I think I can truthfully say I had no idea that motherhood involved so much work. If it wasn't changing the diapers, it was sterilizing the bottles or mixing the formula—and all that screaming, grabbing, crying and upchucking—finally I told Edgar, 'If you don't stop acting like this soon, I won't have any time for Melissa.' "

Third, be flexible in your schedule. For a while your life will be unpredictable. It is often said that "the art of being a good parent is learning to sleep when the baby isn't looking." In a sense that's true. You will be up in the night plus working hard all day. Ideally you should have caught up on your sleep during the last months of pregnancy, but chances are your schedule was so hectic (or your heartburn and the fetal kicking were so intense) that you didn't. Sleep as much as you can now. Be open-minded about your parenting techniques. Don't try to follow books to the letter—including this book! Keep in mind what Lord Rochester (1647–80) once said: "Before I got married I had six theories about bringing up children. Now I have six children and no theories."

Fourth, limit your activities during the first weeks home. Don't try to get everything done—the thank-you notes for baby gifts can wait a while. Politely suggest to friends and neighbors that they come to visit a few weeks from now when you and the baby are more settled in. Don't try to resume an active social calendar immediately. Take a few naps during the day to make up for the interrupted nights. (When you are a new parent you realize that people who say they sleep like a baby usually don't have one.)

It should go without saying that the weeks immediately after your baby is born are most definitely not appropriate for major life changes, like moving or redecorating. Incredibly, however, poor planning results in such events coinciding: "I got home from the hospital one rainy Tuesday morning," said a mother who explained to me that she had her baby exactly 17½ days ago. "I walked in to find the painter, telephone man, plumber, carpenter, and interior decorator all at work. I couldn't even get into bed because it was piled with books and things. It was like a nightmare. 'Depressed' would be a mild way of describing my condition for those first days at home."

Fifth, don't have unrealistic expectations. It does take some time for maternal—and paternal—love to develop. As mentioned earlier, and will be elaborated on in the next section, you will continue to have some mixed feelings. You do have a whole previous life behind you. Before the baby arrived, you did have other commitments and interests—your job, spouse, hobbies—and they are not going to, or should not, disappear now. There is no reason to consider yourself an inadequate parent if you don't turn 100 percent of yourself over to the baby.

Sixth, now that you are parents it's time to get life back to a new type of normal.

Again, probably more than any other factor, it will be fatigue in both of you that will interfere most with the two of you getting reacquainted. This is another important point to consider when evaluating the pros and cons of getting help in the first few weeks.

When you get home from the hospital, take some time to do something nice for the two of you. Have a bottle of special wine at one of your first dinners at home. Ask a trusted friend or relative to come in during that first week so that you can go out to a restaurant, perhaps even see a play or movie. Get out! Reestablish yourselves as a couple, as opposed to only being parents. Of course you'll want, both individually and together, to spend a great deal of time with the baby. But don't ignore your own relationship.

Seventh, remember that postpartum depression can affect both parents. Be understanding of each other and the different types of strains you are both experiencing. Together—and with some outside help with the baby—the chances are you can beat the "after-baby blues."

Parental Bonding

"When I got home from the hospital," Judy, a 29-year-old, first-time mother told me, "all my friends asked me, 'Are you bonding?' I really didn't know what they were talking about. When they explained it to me, I began to worry if something was wrong with me. I didn't know if I was experiencing the feelings they referred to. I've always associated the word 'mother' with marvelous things: love, warmth, kindness, devotion, patience. And now I'm one of those, despite the fact that some days I feel no more motherly than an incubator."

"Bonding" refers to the feeling of motherliness/fatherliness or attachment that grows between a parent and child. It, like parenting generally, is largely a form of learned behavior. As we have already discussed, you should not necessarily expect any surge of feelings or even a strong attachment to your child right away. It can take some time. Research on human childrearing strongly suggests that there is a certain type of "attachment" period that occurs immediately after birth when the mother is emotionally ready to get to know her newborn. Now whether this means that mothers who "room in" with their infants, spending more time with them in the first two or three days, "bond" better than do those who see their babies only three times a day, is not known. When asked about this point, specifically how the bond can be formed in the hospital when mother and baby are separated by the hospital nursery, Dr. Mitzi L. Duxbury, Director of Health Personnel Development at the National Foundation-March of Dimes, responded: "Women who have gone through prepared childbirth usually become acquainted with their babies right after delivery. The mothers are usually awake and aware when the doctor places the newborn on his mother's stomach. Also, many hospitals now have arrangements for mother and baby to share the same room, or they will bring the baby to the mother when she asks to see the infant. And those mothers who see their newborn only at feeding time can make the most of this time by holding him close, singing, talking to, and cuddling the child. Parents who are separated from their infants because of prematurity, low birth weight, or critical illness are encouraged by doctors and nurses to visit the intensive care nursery often, to touch, talk to, cuddle, feed, and help care for the child."

Of course, fathers get acquainted with their infants in the same manner—touching, looking at, and caring for the baby. Whether it is called "mothering," "fathering," "bonding," or "parenting," it is important for all babies to early develop warm, secure, and tender relationships with their parents. But you don't have to approach this scientifically. You really don't need a book to help you with this. Simply do what comes naturally—cuddling, kissing, soothing— always remembering that this bonding is not an instant reflex. It is something that may take time and patience to establish.

THE PHYSICAL

As soon as you have had the baby, you will be watched closely, probably in a recovery room, possibly for an hour or two. During the immediate postpartum period there can be sudden swings in blood pressure and other changes in vital signs, onset of infections of the uterus or urinary tract, and other possible complications, so your pulse, temperature, and blood pressure will be frequently checked. For the entire hospital stay your uterus will be constantly kneaded by a variety of nurses who are not only trying to help it back to its nonpregnant state, but are also evaluating its progress in receding. You may have some initial difficulty urinating the first day, particularly if you have had a local anesthetic. You may need some mild pain killers, iron tablets, and possibly some medication such as Ergonovine to help the uterus contract. But other than that, your recovery and resumption of life's activities will most likely be uneventful.

Postpartum Sex

What is the advice here? Check with your physician. A few with a sense of humor will advise, "At least wait until the anesthetic wears off." But most will suggest waiting four to six weeks, postponing sexual intercourse until after the first postpartum examination, although that rule is not really stringent, some doctors acknowledging that three or four weeks for some women is enough of a recovery period.

"I was breast feeding," another new mother commented, "and I was really surprised how sexy that made me feel. And my husband felt the same way."

"Not me," exclaimed another woman when I asked her if breast feeding had this effect on her. "Actually it made me less oriented toward sex. My breasts were large, full, and they leaked. And it was hardly a turn-on for my husband!"

Obviously, as you can tell from the quotes above, there can be many different types of reaction to the question of sex after pregnancy, and how you will react to the resumption. Masters and Johnson closely observed women in their postpartum periods and found that their sex organs did not respond as rapidly or as intensely as usual to sexual stimulation four or five weeks after birth. Their orgasms were shorter and weaker than they were during or before pregnancy. Many women in the first few weeks notice that their vagina is unusually dry and that factor, among others, makes sex difficult.

But despite the observations by Masters and Johnson, and the undeniable physical difficulties there may be, a substantial number of women find that four or five weeks after childbirth their libido is higher than it ever has been in their lives. Perhaps there is a physiological explanation for this. Perhaps, as some women told me, it is the emotional reaction to the birth, one that brings them closer than ever to their husbands, that explains the phenomenon. Maybe it is due to the fact that they abstained for a month or more before the birth and want to make up for lost time.

Certainly the first time you have intercourse, particularly if you had quite a few stitches following the delivery, you'll want to "go easy." "We were very cautious the first time—the way we were the first time we ever had sex," a new mother explained. "I thought it would be terribly painful, but it turned out to be fine."

Two tips might make postpartum sex more enjoyable. Try some type of lubricant (not vaseline; perferably a K-Y type preparation) to compensate for the natural dryness of the vagina at this time. Second, do some exercises to strengthen your PC muscles (pubococcygal) surrounding the part of the vagina which lost some of its elasticity during the birth. Like other muscles it requires exercise to regain its tone. Exercise it by pretending you are attempting to stop the flow of urine. Tighten the muscle, then relax it.

Successful Breast Feeding

There really is only one useful, constructive tip on successful breast feeding: Relax.

The baby's suckling stimulates the milk production more than anything else. The suckling releases the hormone oxytocin into the blood stream, causing tiny muscles around the milk sacs in the breast to contract and release milk. And this process can be inhibited by any type of anxiety or fatigue. Relax, get comfortable, and you are well on your way to the rewarding experience of breast feeding.

Early in the game you'll probably want to make sure the baby doesn't suck more than a minute at the most on each breast, as his chewing reflex might make the nipple sore, preventing milk flow later. If your breasts become engorged the third or fourth day after delivery, don't be too concerned. This is partly due to the beginning of heavy milk production and partly due to the swelling of breast tissue itself. It will subside on its own, although applying dry or wet heat—a heating blanket or wet towel—might provide some immediate relief. Eventually, the breasts soften, the pain lessens, and the milk becomes thicker and more plentiful. If the baby doesn't seem particularly interested in suckling the first day or two, don't panic and worry that "he's not getting enough to eat." Newborn babies are often not particularly hungry. By the time the colostrum—the thin, sticky, colorless fluid—changes to milk, his appetite will have improved.

Relax—that's the key. Don't worry unnecessarily about your diet. Just eat sensibly, following the basic nutritional guidelines of balance, variety, and moderation. You need plenty of liquid—though not necessarily lots of milk—and a substantial amount of protein and calcium in your diet. But you needn't be fanatical about it. You'll want to avoid drugs other than those prescribed by your doctor and go easy on alcoholic beverages (though a drink or two a day won't harm the child, as long as it doesn't make you dizzy enough to lose your balance!). As always, cigarette smoking is discouraged, now if only because you have the responsibility for a new life and will certainly not want to assume the momentous risks—heart disease; cancer of the lung, bladder, mouth, and other sites; emphysema; accidental fires—which accompany cigarette smoking.

The After-Pregnancy Diet

Given the enormous changes in your anatomy and physiology occurring over the past forty weeks, it's no wonder that you feel a bit different than you did before you started the pregnancy. Right after the birth, especially if you have received anesthetics, you may have some difficulty urinating, possibly resulting from the pressure the baby puts on the bladder as it passes through the birth canal. Constipation is a characteristic complaint of new mothers, generally relieved by gentle laxatives in the first few days. The soreness of the episiotomy may be noticeable for a few days, relieved by anesthetic lotions, sprays, shallow warm baths, heat lamps, and, if necessary, pain-reducing pills (One woman complained to me that her doctor left more stitches in her than there are in an entire knit dress.)

But the physical problem that concerns you most at this point is very likely the question of how you are going to get back in shape. What is most unsettling is, while you expected to be footloose and fanny-free a few days after your return from the hospital, a neighbor sees you and, looking tentatively at your abdomen, asks, "Have you had your baby yet?"

For many women, the extra pounds that linger on after the baby is born are enough in themselves to initiate an acute attack of postpartum depression.

The depressing news is that the extra pounds simply do not come off immediately after you deliver. Generally, you can count on losing about 11 pounds as soon as the baby is born (7½ for the baby, 1½ for the placenta and membranes, 2 for the amniotic fluid) and another 7 or so pounds in the next 12 days (accounted for by accumulated water in your body tissues, the increased weight of the uterus and breasts, and increased blood volume). But from then on, you're on your own. The only way you are going to return to your normal weight—or perhaps even do better than that, taking this opportunity to shed even more extra pounds—is by going on an after-pregnancy diet.

What type of diet is appropriate for a woman who's just had a baby? Obviously, if you are planning to breast feed, no low calorie diet is recommended. Your physician will be recommending a high protein menu with somewhat more calories than he recommended during gestation. But if you are bottle feeding—or have recently terminated breast feeding—you need a high energy, well-balanced, low calorie diet which is based on the Basic Four food categories: the *meat/protein group*, which includes all meats, poultry, fish, eggs, and legumes such as dried beans, peas, and nuts, all of which are good sources of protein and all of which, in addition, supply vitamins of the B complex such as thiamin, riboflavin, niacin, B_6 and B_{12}, and the mineral iron; the *milk group*, products which supply more calcium per serving than any other food, in addition to protein, many of the B vitamins, and vitamins A and D; the *fruit and vegetable group*, to ensure that you are getting enough of vitamins A and C, fiber, minerals, folic acid, and carbohydrates; and the *bread and cereal group*, valuable sources of carbohydrates, protein, thiamin, riboflavin, niacin, and iron. As a general rule, your after-pregnancy diet should consist of 5 ounces from the meat group, 2 servings from the milk category, 4 from fruits and vegetables, and 2–4 from bread and cereal.

But in addition to following good nutritional guidelines and watching calories during the after-birth period, you'll want to enjoy your mealtimes, too. The early days of parenthood are a very special time, and there *is* room in an effective after-pregnancy diet for some leeway: for example, a glass of wine with dinner and a cocktail on weekends—or, if you don't drink alcohol, for an extra special dessert or hors d'oeuvres.

Some Tips for After-Pregnancy Dieting

- No matter how eager you are to return to your regular dress size, *don't* be taken in by one of the many fad diets that are now being promoted. Beware particularly of the low carbohydrate versions. Right after you've had your baby, you need all the energy you can muster up. If you severely restrict carbohydrates, not only will you be embarking on an ineffective long-term solution to your weight problem, but you'll be inviting trouble. You need carbohydrates to provide the "brain food" to keep you going, and if you are following the baby's schedule, that means you'll need your energy both day and night.

- If you are choosing carefully from the Basic Four, you don't need any special vitamin supplements in the postpartum period. But if you do have some prenatal vitamins left over, your physician may recommend that you keep taking them until your supply is used up, just in case your attempts at calorie restriction lead to a slightly unbalanced nutrient intake.

- As soon as you decide to fight your fat, stock up on calorie-saving food—skim milk, cottage cheese, plain yogurt, fresh fruits and vegetables (fill in here with frozen and canned varieties if your favorites are now out of season); and try some of the imitation products—margarines, mayonnaise, gelatin desserts—which offer great caloric savings over their "real" counterparts.

- Increase your normal intake of fruits and vegetables and other high fiber foods to ensure that you are not bothered by constipation, a problem which frequently affects women in the first postpartum months.

- Beware of the middle-of-the-night-snacking syndrome. Just because your baby needs to be fed at 2 A.M. doesn't mean that you have to eat, too. If you fear that opening the refrigerator to get the formula will prove simply irresistible to you, have it well stocked with "free foods" like carrots, celery, cucumbers, and tomatoes.

- Make an effort to cut back on your portions—put half as much as you usually would on your plate. You may be pleasantly surprised about how satiated you feel with smaller amounts of food.

- Don't be overly enthusiastic about supplementing your after-pregnancy diet with vigorous exercises. Check with your doctor before you begin any postpartum exercise program. Chances are he'll want you to take it easy for at least six weeks.

- Take a critical look at your husband's weight! It is not uncommon for the dietary splurges of your pregnancy to affect him, too. If he is overweight, he, too, may benefit from the after-pregnancy diet.

- Most important, accept the fact that you are no longer pregnant. You have no reason for deluding yourself anymore. You may have been eating for two for nine months, but for the next few months, if you want to return to your regular weight, you are going to have to eat for less than one.

Epilogue

A few chapters ago I told you of my own dilemma about whether or not to have children, and alluded to some of the emotional upheaval of our own pregnancy experience. I began this book on a personal note and would like to end it in a similar way.

I first became aware that my pregnancy experience had begun while I was on a publicity tour for my book *A Baby? . . . Maybe*. One morning in a hotel room as I prepared to go on the television program "A.M. Chicago" to discuss whether or not I was going to have a baby, I felt about as nauseous as a seasick ocean voyager. Fortified by five glasses of ginger ale, gripping the arm of the chair, and taking in deep breaths between questions, I managed, without throwing up, to explain to about two million Midwesterners why my husband and I were in a psychological quandary about the pros and cons of parenthood—without revealing the fact that we had actually made our decision a couple of months earlier and that the results of that decision were soon to be very obvious.

My pregnancy experience ended with me exhausted and exhilarated at New York University Hospital when our 8-pound, 2-ounce daughter was placed on my stomach.

In between there was turmoil: fears (particulary early on about having a miscarriage. As the author of a book on the subject, I waited until I was well beyond my third month before I told anyone outside my immediate family. Wouldn't it be awful, I thought, if after bringing all this attention to my dilemma, it was finally resolved, only to end in tragedy. Later on my fears focused on the possibility of multiple births, having become convinced that after asking so many questions I'd be blessed with three or more at once); worries (particularly about how I was going to keep my professional life intact after the baby was born without sacrificing an emotional bond with our child); conflict (my husband was not enthusiastic about the possibility of joining me in the labor or delivery room. When the time came, he was with me during labor and watched his daughter's birth through a glass door—an alternative which, although not right for everyone, was for him and perhaps others); self-doubts ("Why am I not bursting with enthusiasm?" I would constantly ask myself throughout pregnancy. "What if I'm a terrible mother?").

And there were thrills too (my husband's proud Christmas dinner announcement to his family that we were to be parents); rewards (the first time that he, too, could feel the movement of our child); the wonder (that after this was all over, a real-life baby would emerge. I had a sonogram during the middle trimester and carried this "baby picture" with me wherever I went, pointing out the head, torso, limbs); excitement of late pregnancy (despite my lingering fears that "something could go wrong" we couldn't quell the feeling of anticipation we had the day the crib, chest of drawers, and changing table were set up in the baby's room).

At first I thought my ups and downs were unique, ones which only I and perhaps a few other emotionally confused women had to deal with. I know now, of course, that all prospective parents—but particularly those of us who had postponed having children in favor of careers—have these feelings. In the course of talking with men and women, almost all of whom were over 21, I have often wondered how teenagers could survive the emotional turmoil of pregnancy, which invariably coincided with the difficult-enough transition to adulthood.

As I began to write *The Pregnancy Experience*, I accepted the premise—one learned from personal experience—that the key elements in a successful pregnancy, labor, and childbirth are fourfold: First, get all the facts, making sure you have a realistic advance awareness of what to expect. Second, keep an open mind—and a sense of humor. There generally is more than one acceptable way of doing things. Styles and fads come and go but shouldn't dictate your decision. Consider your options. Third, communicate—with your husband, friends, relatives, and, most important, with yourself. Fourth, enjoy every moment! Don't keep waiting for this or that portion of pregnancy to be over. Each has its own thrills and rewards if you take time to identify and develop them.

Now, having completed *The Pregnancy Experience*, I realize that these four guidelines apply as well to the entire course of parenthood, starting with the day of birth. Particularly the first few months of parenthood can be rough and trying for even the most organized, rested, energetic people. Meet the challenge! First, supply yourself with facts. There are a number of excellent guides to growth and development (T. Berry Brazelton's book, *Mothers and Infants; The*

First Twelve Months of Life, edited by Frank Caplan; *The Magic Years,* by Selma Freiberg; *Babyhood,* by Penelope Leach. Keep up with your child's development and also take note of what these books, and magazines like *American Baby,* have to say about the early days of mothering and fathering. Instead of complaining that "you don't know anything about babies," do something about it. Make time in your day to read, even if it means your husband reads half the book, you the other, and you share information.

Second, be open-minded. Many self-appointed childrearing experts may tell you there is only one way ("Don't pick the baby up if s/he cries"; "Only feed him according to schedule"). Read what a number of these "authorities" have to say, talk to your pediatrician, and ultimately use your own good sense—and decide for yourself. And keep a sense of humor! There is a proverb that only two things go away if you ignore them: snow and adolescence. You might add to that list the trying times when your baby cries and cries for no discernible reason.

Third, communicate! Instead of snapping at each other because you're exhausted, discuss your weariness and either postpone tasks or get some help. If you're feeling low, having doubts, or simply need some practical information, talk to friends and relatives about their early weeks of parenthood. You'll probably find that they are pleased to have the opportunity to share their thoughts and experiences with you.

Finally, enjoy the first weeks of your baby's life! Everyone will tell you how those days disappear so quickly. By the time your child is six months old you will know what they mean. (We often find ourselves saying to our daughter, "Slow down! We haven't read that chapter of the books yet!") It is trite, but he or she is not going to stay a baby very long. Save some time for talking, playing, cuddling, teaching. This is at least as important as sterilized bottles, formula, and clean, dry diapers.

Your pregnancy experience is over, but a new, equally exciting phase of your life has begun. You are about to experience the joy of rediscovering the world, reliving things you have long forgotten. (How long has it been since you became fascinated watching an ant crawl up a blade of grass? When is the last time someone asked you

why she couldn't take a bath in the dishwasher, what makes the vac-
uum cleaner work, and what the opposite of yellow is?) Grow with
your child. Take advantage of every moment. Make the sequel to a
rewarding, enjoyable pregnancy experience a life enriched by the
presence of this new human being you created together.

Selected References

References marked with an asterisk (*) are recommended background reading for the prepregnancy, pregnancy, and early parenthood periods.

*American Baby magazine, 1967–1978.

"Antenatal Battering." British Medical Journal, December 1974.

Anthony, E., and T. Benedek. Parenthood: Its Psychology and Psychopathology. Boston: Little, Brown and Company, 1970.

Arms, S. Immaculate Deception: A New Look at Women and Childbirth in America. New York: Bantam, 1977.

*Baby Talk magazine, 1975–1978.

*Barber, V. and M. Skaggs. The Mother Person. New York: Bobbs-Merrill, 1975.

Barclay, R., and M. Barclay. "Aspects of the Normal Psychology of Pregnancy: The Mid-Trimester." American Journal of Obstetrics and Gynecology 125 (1976):207.

Bernard, J. The Future of Motherhood. New York: Dial Press, 1964.

Bibring, G., and A. Valenstien, "Psychological Aspects of Pregnancy." Clinical Obstetrics and Gynecology 19 (1976):357.

*Bing, E. Six Practical Lessons for an Easier Childbirth. New York: Bantam Books, 1969.

*Bing, E., and L. Colman. Making Love During Pregnancy. New York: Bantam Books, 1977.

*Boston Children's Medical Center. "Pregnancy, Birth and the Newborn Baby." Boston: Delacorte Press, 1972.

*Brazelton, T. B. *Infants and Mothers: Differences in Development.* New York: Delta Books, 1969.

*Brennan, B., and J. R. Heilman. *The Complete Book of Midwifery.* New York: Dutton, 1977.

Brody, J. E. "How a Mother Affects Her Unborn Baby." *Woman's Day* reprint (1970) issued by the Office of Research Reporting, National Institute of Child Health and Human Development, National Institute of Health, Bethesda, Maryland 20014.

*Caplan, F. *The First Twelve Months of Life.* New York: Grosset and Dunlap, 1973.

Carty, E. "My, You're Getting Big." *The Canadian Nurse,* August 1970.

Clark, A., and R. Hale. "Sex During and After Pregnancy." *American Journal of Nursing* 74 (1974):1430.

Colman, A. "Psychological State During First Pregnancy." *American Journal of Orthopsychiatry* 36 (July 1969):4.

*Colman, A. and L. *Pregnancy: The Psychological Experience.* New York: Herder and Herder, 1971.

Curley, J., *et al. The Balancing Act: A Career and a Baby.* Chicago: Chicago Review Press, 1976.

Curtis, J. *Working Mothers.* New York: Doubleday, 1976.

Curtis, L., and Y. Coroles. *Pregnant and Lovin' It.* Tucson, Arizona: H. P. Boox, 1977.

David, V. *Father's Doing Nicely.* New York: Bobbs-Merrill, 1938.

De Beauvoir, S., *The Second Sex.* New York: Vintage Books, 1974.

Deutsch, H., *The Psychology of Women* (Vol. II, *Motherhood*). New York: Bantam, 1973.

*Dick-Read, G. *Childbirth Without Fear.* 2nd ed. New York: Harper and Row, 1959.

Dodson, Fitzhugh. *How to Father.* New York: New American Library, 1974.

Erickson, M. "The Relationship Between Psychological Variables and Specific Complications of Pregnancy, Labor and Delivery." *Journal of Psychosomatic Research* 20 (1976):207.

Expecting magazine, 1975–.

Fallaci, O. *Letter to a Child Never Born.* New York: Simon and Schuster, 1975.

Fawcett, J. *Psychology and Population.* The Population Council, 1970.

Fielding, W. *Pregnancy: The Best State of the Union.* New York: T. Y. Crowell Company, 1971.

*Fraiberg, S. *The Magic Years: Understanding and Handling the Problems of Early Childhood.* New York: Scribner and Sons, 1959.

Geissler, J. "Motherhood: A Time for Letting Go." *Redbook,* March 1975.

Gillman, R. "The Dreams of Pregnant Women and Maternal Adaptation." *American Journal of Orthopsychiatry* 38 (1968):688.

Gordon, R. "Factors in Postpartum Emotional Adjustment." *Obstetrics and Gynecology* 25 (1965):158.

*Group for the Advancement of Psychiatry. *The Joys and Sorrows of Parenthood.* New York: Charles Scribner's Sons, 1973.

Gunn, A. "The Normal Pregnancy." *Nursing Times,* January 15, 1970.

*Guttmacher, A. *Pregnancy, Birth and Family Planning.* New York: Signet, 1973.

Hogenboom, P. "Man in Crisis: The Father." *Journal of Psychiatric Nursing,* Sept–Oct., 1967, p. 457.

Hollender, M. and J. McGehee. "The Wish to Be Held During Pregnancy." *Journal of Psychosomatic Research* 18 (1974):193.

Horowitz, M., and N. Horowitz. "Psychologic Effects of Education for Childbirth." *Psychosomatics* 8 (1967):196.

Hott, J. R. "The Crisis of Expectant Fatherhood." *American Journal of Nursing* 76 (1976):1436.

Hunt, D., *Parents and Children in History.* New York: Basic Books, 1970.

Jarrahi-Zadeh, A., *et al.* "Emotional and Cognitive Changes in Pregnancy and Early Puerperium." *British Journal of Psychiatry* 115 (1969):797.

Kotchek, L. "Now I've Been There." *American Journal of Nursing* 72 (1972):1247.

Lazarre, J. *The Mother Knot.* New York: Dell, 1976.

Leach, P. *Babyhood.* New York: Knopf, 1976.

LeMasters, E. W. "Parenthood as Crisis," in *Crises Intervention.* New York: H. J. Parad, Family Services Association, 1974.

Lerner, B. "On the Need to Be Pregnant." *International Journal of Psychoanalysis* 48 (1967):288.

Light, H., and C. Fenster. "Maternal Concerns During Pregnancy." *American Journal of Obstetrics and Gynecology* 118 (1974):46.

*McBride, A. B. *The Growth and Development of Mothers.* New York: Harper and Row, 1973.

McCauley, C. S. *Pregnancy After 35.* New York: Dutton, 1976.

McKinlay, J. "The Sick Role—Illness and Pregnancy." *Social Science and Medicine* 6 (1972):561.

Mead, M. *Blackberry Winter.* New York: Simon and Schuster, 1972.

Meikle, S., and R. Gerritse. "A Comparison of Husband-Wife Responses to Pregnancy." *Journal of Psychology* 83 (1973):17.

Meyer, H. "What Parents Worry About in Their Newborn Infants." *Medical Times* 100 (1972):51.

Milinaire, C. *Birth*. New York: Harmony Books, 1974.

Morton, M. D. *Pregnancy Notebook*. New York: Workman Publishing, 1972.

Nadelson, C., *et al*. "The Pregnant Therapist." *American Journal of Psychiatry* 131 (1974):1107.

National Institute of Child Health and Human Development. "Antenatal Diagnosis and Down's Syndrome." DHEW Publication 74:548, United States Government Printing Office, 1973.

Palmer, R. L. "A Psychosomatic Study of Vomiting of Early Pregnancy." *Journal of Psychosomatic Research* 17 (1973):303.

Panter, G., and S. M. Linde. *Now That You've Had Your Baby*. New York: Spectrum Books, 1977.

Parker, E. *The Seven Ages of Women*. Baltimore: The Johns Hopkins Press, 1960.

Pines, D. "Pregnancy and Motherhood: Interaction Between Fantasy and Reality." *British Journal of Medical Psychology* 45 (1972):333.

Price, J. *You're Not Too Old to Have a Baby*. New York: Farrar, Straus, Giroux, 1977.

Rheingold, J. C. *The Fear of Being a Woman*. New York: Grune and Stratton, 1964.

Rich, A. *Of Women Born: Motherhood as an Experience and Institution*. New York, W. W. Norton, 1976.

Richardson, S., and A. Guttmacher, eds. *Childbearing: Its Social and Psychological Aspects*. Baltimore: The Williams and Wilkins Company, 1967.

Robin, A. "The Psychological Changes of Normal Parturition." *Psychiatric Quarterly* 36 (1962):129.

Rubin, R. "Cognitive Style in Pregnancy." *American Journal of Nursing*, March 1970.

Salk, L. *Preparing for Parenthood*. New York: McKay, 1974.

Schaefer, G. *The Expectant Father: A Practical Guide*. New York: Barnes and Noble, 1972.

Solberg, D., *et al*. "Sexual Behavior in Pregnancy." *New England Journal of Medicine* 288 (1973):1098.

Stone, A. "Cues to Interpersonal Distress Due to Pregnancy." *American Journal of Nursing*, November 1965.

Tolor, A., and P. DiGrazia. "Sexual Attitudes and Behavior Patterns During and Following Pregnancy." *Archives of Sexual Behavior* 5 (1976):539.

*Whelan, E. M. *A Baby? . . . Maybe: A Guide to Making the Most Fateful Decision of Your Life*. New York: Bobbs-Merrill, 1975.

———. Boy or Girl? The Sex Selection Technique That Makes All Others Obsolete. New York: Bobbs-Merrill, 1977.

"Willful Exposure to Unwanted Pregnancy." *Canadian Medical Association Journal* 111 (1974):1945.

Yamamoto, K., and D. Kinney. "Pregnant Women's Ratings of Different Factors Influencing Psychological Stress During Pregnancy." *Psychological Reports* 39 (1976):203.

Zimmerman, K. "The Public Health Nurse and Emotions of Pregnancy." *Public Health Nurse* 39 (1947):63.

Index